the losses
we keep

the losses we keep

OUR JOURNEY OF FERTILITY, LOSS, AND NEVER-ENDING HOPE

JAMI CRIST

AND OTHER CONTRIBUTING AUTHORS

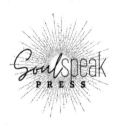

Soulspeak
PRESS

Published and distributed by Soul Speak Press
Virginia, USA

Library of Congress Control Number: 2024917233
Crist, Jami
The Losses We Keep: Our Journey of Fertility, Loss and Never-Ending Hope
ISBN: 978-1-958472-11-8 (Paperback)
ISBN: 978-1-958472-12-5 (eBook)

To our Spirit Babies,
Thank you for changing us into the mothers we didn't know
we needed to be. This is written for you.

CONTENTS

INTRODUCTION

If you're picking up this book, most likely the title resonated with you because you are going through the experience of a pregnancy loss, IVF, repeatedly finding out you're not getting pregnant and don't know why, or are hitting a standstill in your motherhood journey and you don't know where to turn for help.

Like most women growing up in the late '90s and early '00s, I was taught that even looking at a penis could get me pregnant; no one ever really taught me how my body actually worked nor did they prepare me for where the pregnancy journey could take me. Like so many others, I went to my OB-GYN declaring I was ready to start trying and their advice was simple: "Just come off your birth control and give it a few months." That's it. The indication was that when you're ready to have your baby, it will happen in no time.

Sure, maybe that happens for some women and I am happy for them; but that wasn't the case for my family, and I wasn't remotely prepared or educated on where the alternative path could lead. Now I know, unfortunately, that one in four women miscarry, and eight out of ten miscarriages happen in the first trimester, or before the twelfth week of pregnancy. To be honest, I was utterly oblivious to this. I was proud of my body when I got pregnant so quickly the first time. I quickly shifted my focus to my corporate career because I felt I had something to prove; I needed to show the world that I could do it all. However, life took a significant pivot.

We walked into our sixteen-week ultrasound appointment and were delivered the news that our baby wasn't going to make it. I was completely blindsided; I didn't even realize something like this was possible. We had made it to the twelfth week and everything looked good. We stuck to the twelve-week rule before we started sharing with friends and family. Then, we hit the sixteen-week mark, and everything went wrong very quickly.

The experience of losing our daughter was complicated as we had to have immediate surgery. As I was recovering, I realized I didn't know anyone in my community who had gone through something like this, or at least had shared openly about it. To make things even harder, I had multiple friends who were due with their first babies around the same time as I was supposed to deliver. As their pregnant bellies grew, I grew more empty and alone. I searched social media and scoured the internet for blogs on similar stories of women who had gone through the same thing. I found a few stories of women sharing their heartbreaking news, and I joined a few pregnancy loss groups, but I found myself in a dark hole that spiraled because none of their news was very good. I read the few books I could find that would offer advice about how to cope with a pregnancy loss, but frankly, the messaging was usually too religious for me, and just didn't resonate. I was angry with my Higher Power for doing this to me and my husband.

It seemed no one could tell me how to care for myself physically, how to cope with my body as I gained weight with a belly that was starting to grow but now had nothing to show for it. I was at a loss mentally, physically, and spiritually. What I wanted and needed was a resource that would share real stories about how hard this journey actually was. I needed to feel like someone else understood what I was going through, but could also offer a guiding light to the hope that I would indeed have my baby, someday.

Once I shared our story on social media, I had several friends and strangers reach out to share their own unexpected journey to motherhood—they reminded me I wasn't alone. These women welcomed me into the shittiest club I've ever belonged to, but simultaneoulsy they were my greatest guides on this arduous journey. Many of their stories are the reason I did not give up on having my baby in my arms someday. As I was making my way down my broken path toward motherhood, I promised myself that I would share the gift of solidarity with other women someday; which is what we have done through this book.

In collaboration with eight other women who have survived their own difficult journeys toward motherhood, we bring you our offering, *The Losses We Keep*. This title is so resonant because no matter the number of babies some of us hold in our arms, we hold every single loss in our hearts. We know, just like you, that the loss of a baby does not go away, despite the healing we may have experienced. As you head down your own path of healing, we want you to know, more than anything, that YOU ARE NOT ALONE! This book is meant to help you understand this crucial truth; we want you to hold our stories close to your heart. As you go through the stories in this collection, we want you to be reminded that you are in good company. Through these pages you will meet some of the strongest, most resilient women. They have been forced to walk this path, and might still be on it, but they have chosen to share their stories because they want you to know this critically important truth: They see you and are here with you for as long as it takes. We know from experience that no one gets it until they go through it. These members get it. And they welcome you into this club with open and loving arms.

We are standing with you and are sending you love. Thank you for allowing us to walk with you on this journey and share our hearts with you.

With love and hope,

Jami

RUNNING SHOES

Jami Crist

I pulled into the parking spot outside of my new therapist's office. It was the first time I had ever gone to therapy, and I was nervous. *Do I really need a therapist?*

"I can't believe I am actually doing this," I said aloud to no one as I looked in the visor mirror, in an attempt to pull myself together after crying the whole way there. I looked out my window and watched as raindrops spattered in uneven patterns on the glass and then slid down. It was a dreary day at the end of October. Typically, October was my favorite as I had claimed it as my birthday month. It was a fun joke between me and my husband Brad. But this October was very different.

It's like the sky is crying for me too. I looked back into the mirror and addressed my reflection with maternal authority: "I will just go to this one appointment, and that's it. No pressure." I still felt guilty for leaving work in the middle of the day to go to therapy, which, looking back, is ridiculous. I had just lost my baby and had every right to take time off and care for my mental health. Because I didn't know how this whole therapy thing worked, I let myself cry on the drive up so I could release the tears in private; I didn't want my new therapist to see me cry. After fruitless attempts to dry my blotchy face, I finally felt put together enough to walk into the office. As soon as I walked through the door, I noticed something different. There was a stick of palo santo burning at reception, and the smoke was wafting through the air. The books that lined her shelves weren't thick psychology textbooks but paperbacks explaining the modalities of breathwork, how the body is affected by trauma, and how the universe has your back.

Hmmm . . . this is different than I expected. . . . I couldn't decide if I felt comforted by the environment, or more nervous. A shorter woman with brown hair came around the corner and greeted my name just as I started to introduce myself. I laughed nervously as I stuck my hand out to shake hers, and was even more surprised when she ignored my hand and came in for a massive hug instead.

Not your typical therapist, I mused. Still mystified by our initial encounter, I took a seat on her couch; my body tightened as soon as I made contact with the fabric.

"What brought you in today, Jami?" Mary Ann asked, staring at me directly in the eyes as she sat relaxed in her comfy looking chair.

I took a deep breath and dived in. I explained that only two weeks ago, I had been sixteen weeks pregnant when we found out the baby wasn't going to make it due to a condition called arthrogryposis. I told her about the D&C, my voice breaking when I got to the part about needing to have my baby removed from my body on my birthday. "I'm not surprised this happened . . . because I feel like my path always had to be a tough one," I explained bleakly. "But I had a friend that mentioned you helped her when she lost her baby at six months . . . and well, I don't know. . . ." My voice trailed off as I did my best to hold back the tears. I focused my gaze on my running shoes, briefly wondering why I had paired them with my skirt.

"Ugh, Jami, I am so sorry to hear this. This is heartbreaking, and it's a lot. How are you taking care of yourself as you grieve the loss of your baby?" Mary Ann's face was full of compassion and she waited patiently, completely comfortable with the sadness that had taken a seat on the couch next to me. With her next question, she invited all the other emotions in. "And did he or she have a name?"

My heart tore a little when I thought about the name. "It was going to be a girl, and we already had a name picked out. It was going to be Callie Joy." I rushed on because thinking about the name was too painful to linger on.

"I am doing okay." Ever the survivor, as the words came out of my mouth, I knew it wasn't true. My body wanted to say something else, to tell the real story, but it simply didn't know how. "I am back at work this week and will teach my cycle classes again this weekend. I think that's good. I am ready to move forward, and that's what I'm doing." My words felt hollow as I felt the couch buzzing from the vibration of my phone. The itch to check it, because I was anxious about missing something from work, felt almost uncontrollable. I was powerless as the restless energy took over my body; sweat began beading on my legs under my skirt.

Mary Ann nodded as she sat back in her chair and asked more follow up questions, "Who's supporting you during this time as you grieve the loss of your daughter?"

I looked back down at my shoes and ticked off the list. "My husband, my aunt, who's like a mom to me, and my other family and friends. My mom isn't around; she passed away just about two years ago."

The thought of not having a "normal" family to support me during this time stirred up haunting memories from my tumultuous childhood. I was familiar with this reality. I'd had a rough start, and I believed that my life might never be easy; that I was undeserving of easy. "Normal" could never be a state I lived in. I loathed myself for not being nurturing enough because of how I was raised. Maybe that's why my baby died—I had been abandoned by my mother and now, it seemed, by my unborn baby.

A flashback to my nine-year-old self emerged as I continued to work out what to say to Mary Ann next. In my mind's eye, I could clearly see a little girl who desperately wanted to feel loved by her mother; she wanted to be tucked into bed by her parents, parents who showed up to her softball games and told her they were proud of her accomplishments. This need to belong and feel normal was deeply entrenched by the second grade, where I attempted to change my last name from Gobao to Scuse. Everyone else in the classroom had the same last name as their parents, and so I wanted that too.

At the age of five, my aunt and uncle had become my legal guardians. And while everyone else had a mom and dad at home, I would sit next to the window at my aunt and uncle's, my little face pressed up against the glass, waiting for my mom to pull up on her visiting days. My aunt never explained why she didn't show up—I got used to it and never held it against her. She was an alcoholic with a disease.

As I grew older, I embraced the belief that I wasn't good enough for my mom to want to change so she could be with me. It was a belief that turned into a hard fact and would be the force that propelled me to achieve well into adulthood.

"Can you tell me more about your mom, babe?" Mary Ann asked, pulling me from my troubled memories and back into the present.

I explained that I loved my mom, but we had a challenging relationship. I told her about her alcoholism and how we had lost my dad when I was four. I told her about my first memories of going to live with my aunt, who had legal guardianship over me. My mom, the life of the party, could never let the party end. I had always felt like the adult in the relationship, and, while I loved her very much, that was hard.

A tear escaped my control and ran down my face as I told Mary Ann about my mom dying, one week after I got married in December 2017. A sob caught in my throat as I remembered that unexpected call telling me she was gone. Just when things were shifting, getting better, it was all over. "We never got to really enjoy our next chapter together. It was too late." I could feel the pit in my stomach grow deeper, and my eyes, no matter how hard I blinked, couldn't stop the swell of tears. I apologized for crying in her office.

"Why do you keep running, Jami?" I wiped a tear from my cheek and pulled a tissue from the sofa table in front of me, frowning in confusion.

"I'm not sure I know what you mean?"

She shifted in her chair and leaned forward, ready to dig a little deeper into my story. In that moment, I realized there was so much more to unpack.

"Well, the way I see it, you haven't even grieved the loss of your mom, and now you have to mourn the passing of your baby. That's hard." She paused to let those words sink in.

"It feels like this baby came into your life for a reason. So, why do you keep running?"

I shook my head, unable to understand why she thought I was running from it all. I was here in therapy, wasn't I? I had walked in . . . sort of willingly. I told her what had happened; *I know it fucking sucks, but can't we just then move forward?*

"I've been here before—when hard things happen—and I've made it through." I explained that my path has always felt different from others around me, ever since I was a kid. I demonstrated that I was a planner, a doer, I made things happen. I turned my hardships into fuel—I had loads of proof that I could survive anything. *How can she say I'm running?*

Her question stirred me up. We hit the end of the session, so I avoided answering her question further and reverted to what I knew how to do: show her that I was doing the work to be here.

After the appointment, I hustled to the car so I could get downtown to work. Throughout the drive back to the city, all I could hear was her question, "Why do you keep on running?" In the back of my mind, I could hear just about everyone I knew saying things like, "Jami, you just don't stop" and "I don't know how you do it; you're amazing for all you do" or "You are so strong for what you have overcome." Those compliments were a badge of honor. They were my proof that I was "normal" despite being dealt such a shitty hand. I prided myself on not sleeping, on skipping social events with friends or family because of my "job" responsibilities. It was so important to me to be seen as the hardest working person in the room so I could show my worth. Taking time out of my day to do therapy felt like a heavy lift, but I was doing it. How dare she say I was running?

After that first loss, it was recommended by my acupuncturist to wait three months after my period came back before I tried to get pregnant again. Right before the holiday, my period returned, and I immediately started the three-month countdown. As I opened up my planner to find the month of March to remind myself we could start trying, I noticed March 28 was marked with a heart. The due date of our little girl.

March felt like it took forever to get to. I traveled nonstop all winter for work; Austin, Texas, to Portland, Oregon, and wrapped up in Los Angeles before the world shut down. Now that I had the time to research, plan, and prepare, I convinced my husband that we should start trying again but this time, have lots of planned sex around my ovulation time. He didn't have any complaints about this, like most men who hear that their wife wants to have lots of sex. However, that month changed very quickly because of the COVID-19 shutdown. As many around the world were trying to navigate this stressful time, so too were we—we were concerned about our health; my husband was scrambling to save his company from lack of revenue; and my job-related travel ultimately stopped, and all my time was spent drafting fast pivots to support the business at Under Armour. Add forced sex into the picture, and there wasn't anything romantic about trying to conceive that month.

Spring still sprung during that COVID year, even though it felt like the world was still on hold. Then came summer, and the first anniversary of our first positive pregnancy test. Scrolling through my phone, I lost many hours to fantasizing and remembering the same time last year; my scroll stopped on the photo of my positive pregnancy test. When I took the photo, I immediately sent it to my aunt with a surprised face emoji. Hoping to catch her off guard and surprise her, it did just that. And now, a year later, I wasn't pregnant, even though we had been trying since March, and we were around that five-month mark of nothing happening. The doctors recommended seeing a specialist if nothing happened within six months of trying. But sure enough, just as we were approaching that six-month mark, I had the double blue lines show up giving me a positive pregnancy test. I immediately called Brad, bursting with excitement, "Babe, we did it! We're pregnant!" I screamed into the phone. He laughed in surprised response.

I immediately opened up the What to Expect app on my phone to plug in that we had conceived so I could calculate our due date: April 2021. I immediately called the doctor to get blood work done in order to ensure my hCG levels were showing I was pregnant and scheduled my first ultrasound, but this time, I wanted to do it earlier because I just couldn't wait to see a heartbeat. I looked at the calendar in my planner: *okay, at seven weeks, I can go in.* It would be right after I got back from my cousin's wedding.

We arrived in Connecticut on Labor Day weekend, ready to celebrate my cousin's nuptials. I woke up early to get my morning run in before I had to help set up and prepare for the event. I took a scenic route along a back road that I wasn't familiar with, but was tracking to ensure I could get back to the hotel in one piece. It was getting humid, and I was really sweating, so I took my shirt off, admiring my stomach, daydreaming about this baby in me. As I kept my pace, I stroked my belly with my hands trying to make a connection. We were together, running and moving as one.

Running was something I loved doing during my first pregnancy; I felt like it was "our time" together and was determined to keep up that practice during this pregnancy. I returned from my run and hurried up to get in the shower to prepare for the ceremony.

As I peeled off my sticky clothes, I turned the tap on to get the shower nice and hot. Squatting over the toilet to pee before hopping in the shower, I noticed a stomach cramp, and looked down. The toilet water was an odd shade of pink. I wiped and was horrified to see bright red blood on the paper. A gut-wrenching feeling took over me. *It's just a little blood, that's normal this early on,* I told myself, taking deep breaths, trying to calm down. I wrapped myself in a towel and walked into the room; Brad was relaxing on the bed. Trying to get the words out, I told him there was some blood. We both talked ourselves out of believing that something was wrong. I reached for my phone and immediately went to Doctor Google.

"Okay, okay, it says this is normal," I explained to him. "I am not having full-on bleeding, so I think we're okay." We decided to go to the wedding and just try to enjoy ourselves.

As the night progressed, I grew more nervous as I became increasingly unwell. I obsessively kept checking to make sure blood wasn't coming out onto my dress. Every few minutes I would get up from the table and head to the bathroom to see if there was more blood. When I returned to the table, I tried to keep up with the small talk with my family.

"Jam, come dance with us!" My friends and family were up on the dance floor having such a good time. I waved them off with a laugh and claimed to have had too much to drink to dance without hurting myself. But deep down inside, I knew what was happening. I just didn't want to tell them.

We got back to Baltimore the day after the wedding, and by that evening, my body had progressed into a total miscarriage. We called the doctor on call to see if there was anything else I could do to help the pain until the miscarriage completed; she recommended that I stay home, rest, and drink a lot of water. But other than that, there wasn't anything they could do to help. It was a couple of grueling days, but after I stopped bleeding, I just picked up where I had left off, and buried my head into work or any other distraction that came my way. I just wanted to escape the emptiness I felt inside.

One of the ways I avoided the emptiness and remained in control was by making a plan. As if I were back in my college athlete days training for preseason, I mapped out a pregnancy plan as if I were readying myself for training day. Once my period returned, I got down to business. I marked off on my calendar when my ovulation window would occur and didn't schedule anything with friends after that time because I would be within the two-week waiting window after trying. I was avoiding alcohol, just in case I was pregnant, and I sure as hell wasn't going to ruin any of my chances. I created rules that were meant to protect and control my body, in case it happened. I was careful to mark my planner and review my cycle on the app every morning to ensure I was tracking correctly. I did my research on how to best prepare to get pregnant and determined doing all the food prep recommended for the egg-quality diet was the way to go. I stuffed my Amazon cart with ovulation strips. I scaled back on caffeine and drank bone broth in the mornings because I had read that helped women get pregnant. You name it, I tried it.

My body could get pregnant, this we knew, and that was half the battle. But, there was a chromosome issue every time. With each pregnancy, I would convince myself this was the ONE. But the pregnancy always ended in the doctor's office with an "I am so sorry, we see an issue with the fetus," and then being escorted to the back door of the office so I wouldn't scare the happy pregnant women with my red blotchy face. The third pregnancy loss ended at thirteen weeks in March 2021 due to a condition called triploidy, which can cause a molar pregnancy and cancer. This condition would have led to chemo and being unable to try again for another six months. Still, luckily, our results for a molar pregnancy were negative. So we could start trying again.

After the third loss, we decided to pack up and move to the beach for six weeks, starting at the beginning of the summer. We wanted to do something for us, and the beach was our happy place. It felt more like the great escape out of Baltimore; I could avoid seeing people I would know and run into, and have the excuse to decline the baby shower invites. It was easier to say, "Oh, I am so sorry to miss celebrating you and your expectant bundle of joy, but we will be at the beach!" I got really good at declining invitations, with a fake smile plastered on my face when, deep down, I felt resentment against everyone. Why do they get to have their baby and I don't?

As we were counting down the days to leaving, I found out I was pregnant again in mid-May. It was so quick after our last loss, pregnancy number four. Part of me was so excited to be pregnant as we headed to our haven at the beach. Despite my trepidation, I kept imagining myself lying on the beach in a cute bikini that showcased my little baby bump just so. *It would be so special.* The other part of me didn't want to be excited anymore. I didn't really know how. And then there were "The Rules" I would remind myself of. *Don't get too excited so you don't get disappointed again. Don't get attached this time; that way you won't be as upset if it doesn't work out, Jami.* It was like *Groundhog Day.* Copy and paste the same routine; pulling up the What to Expect app; calculate the due date (mid-January!); call and schedule the OB-GYN for blood work and a scan in seven weeks. The earlier I could get in, the better, so I didn't have to wait in case something went wrong.

We went into the Advanced Fetal Care department at the University of Maryland Medical Center for our scan and stared at the screen. By now, we were seasoned and jaded. I knew what the screen was supposed to look like. The tech regarded us with empathy, but I already knew. "I am very sorry, but it seems like there isn't a fetus." I looked at Brad, and our defeat was mirrored in each other's faces.

"Well, maybe we are still early, and nothing has fully developed yet?" I said this so unconvincingly, even I didn't believe it. With sad, pitiful eyes, the technician explained that there would be a fetus at this point. We left the room and were escorted out the back door of the office—again. This time, there was no ultrasound picture, my hands were as empty as my womb and heart. We got in the car, and I slammed my hands on the leather panel in front of me and screamed, "Goddamn it, I should have known better than to think it would work out this time!" Brad reached over the center consul to hold me as I wept in his arms. We rode home in silence, packed up the car, and went back to the beach; we had to escape again.

I didn't tell anyone. Instead, I gave up. I had failed. And that just wasn't me; I was the go-getter who pursued what I wanted no matter what it took or how hard I had to work. I tried to appear unbothered by the fact that all my friends were pregnant and starting their families. But deep down, I knew I was angry and jealous and felt like I was failing and falling behind. Physically, I kept feeling this sensation, as if my body was giving out, similar to when I approached mile twenty-one along the marathon course during a race. It was always at that point that I would start to doubt myself, my breath would get deeper as I felt the anxiety sink in, my legs would feel like bricks, heavy as I tried to take one step, putting one foot in front of the other, and my hands would tingle. I always wanted to stop, but I could somehow always talk myself into getting to the next mile.

Almost there, Jami. Don't give up. That's how I had been managing, up until this fourth miscarriage.

When it came to a race, I knew there was a finish line. I could see it, and I had control over getting there. But motherhood was proving to be a completely different finish line, and I worried I would never see it. I was growing so angry with my body and in self-preservation, disassociated from it. I didn't even feel like I was in it anymore. My body, four pregnancies later, three surgeries, two miscarriages, was some foreign object that could not bring a pregnancy to full term. One morning I woke up and did the calculations: I had been pregnant for a total of forty-five weeks. That was more than a full-term pregnancy, and I had nothing to show for it besides weight gain and fluctuating hormones that were all over the damn place.

Still, there were no answers from the doctors on why these losses kept happening. I was getting so frustrated with the lack of answers, that I started to raise my voice over the phone with them; I wanted answers! But they had none. "Sometimes, this is what happens," they would tell me. *CEOs can fly to the damn moon for fuck's sake, but we still can't figure out why women can't have a healthy baby? Welcome to women's healthcare in 2021, folks.* I started to shut my friends out because I was jealous of their pregnancies. I even started to question my marriage.

After two attempts of taking misoprostol, my body couldn't pass the pregnancy tissue naturally from the fourth pregnancy. Another D&C surgery was scheduled; this was the third surgery my body was preparing for. I was, again, surrounded by the off-white hospital curtains and sitting on the cold leather chair, stripped down in a hospital gown and oversized gray grippy socks. I walked into the dark surgery room and laid on the cold table, each heel placed into the left and right leg stirrups. The nursing staff reminded me of the oxygen nose tube and placed it into me for the procedure. I put on my headphones to listen to a meditation to cover the background noise of the surgery and talk among the staff about the procedure.

"Okay, Jami, we're going to get started," the doctor told me. I closed my eyes and turned up the sound on my headphones, and tears slowly rolled down my cheek. Uttering the words to myself, "I give up."

I thought to myself, *Maybe this is a sign from the universe that Brad and I aren't supposed to be together because we can't have a child together . . . maybe I'm not supposed to be a mother.* I got to a point where I surrendered. Hands up in the air and lost the will to hold tight to a vision I desperately wanted through these last few years. There was nothing else I could do. I had done everything by the books, and here we were with no baby. As someone who used to be so proud of my body and its strength, as an athlete who could push through the hardest of physical challenges, I grew so angry and hateful towards my body and its lack of ability to maintain a healthy pregnancy. It was devastating.

I woke up one morning and stared in the mirror. Looking back at me was the reflection of a woman I didn't even recognize anymore. She was tired—so tired. Detached, disconnected, barely there. I realized in that moment that my body, mind, and heart were no longer connected, and they wouldn't be for a very long time. But I was in my favorite place in the whole world—the beach—and I knew I needed to try to get back to me. So I surrendered and decided to go out for sushi and a cocktail. To hell with all the rules. I was secretly elated to think about not drinking bone broth first thing in the morning. It was time to enjoy living again—I had a few weeks ahead at the beach, and I would enjoy it and figure out the next step in September.

I convinced Brad that we should start the IVF process in the fall. He didn't love the thought of IVF, but encouraged me to do what was best for me. He would be there. We agreed to take these last few weeks at the beach and live as if nothing mattered. No planning or pushing or trying to conceive a baby. As I sipped my Orange Crush, the boulders of grief, frustration, and disappointment rolled off my back. It felt like true freedom, and for a moment, it was glorious.

During those six weeks away, I woke up early every morning to take my dog down to the beach so he could swim without disturbing beachgoers. It was a shimmer of magic that lit up every day. In all the turmoil and loss, I had forgotten what magic felt like, and what these shimmering moments can do for the soul. I would reflect as I watched the sun hit the water and take a big inhale of the salty sea air. It cleansed and refreshed me in a way that made me feel grounded. As I dug my toes into the sand, I would gaze out onto the water, hoping for a sign from my spirit baby. I would return to the house and do my morning pages, three pages of hand-written, stream-of-consciousness writing, while sipping my coffee, relishing in the heat of the summer mornings. And in those moments, I found peace.

As our time at the beach was ending shortly after the July holiday, during one of my morning page sessions, I stumbled upon a quote by Brené Brown. She said, "When you are uncertain, you feel at risk, you feel exposed, but don't tap out. Stay brave, stay uncomfortable, stay in the cringy moment, and lean into the hard conversation. Stay brave." That resonated with me so deeply. When I looked over my life, I had somehow managed to never tap out.

My childhood was hard, but I was better for it. I had known this for a while. It made me who I am today. And while my life had never been this perfect linear line, I had ended up pretty okay, and things had worked out somehow, someway. I remembered the complicated conversation I had forced myself to have with my high school sweetheart and long term boyfriend. My gut knew I wanted something else, and even though it was scary and hard, I had leaned in. It was hard AF, but things worked out for the best, because then, I met my husband.

And then I reflected over the time I had decided to transfer to a new college after my freshman year because I wasn't happy there. I had the conversations to make the change, and I know I wouldn't be the woman I am today if I hadn't leaned in and made that change. I had figured out how to be brave then. So, why couldn't I be brave now? Once I realized I had options, my gut did what it always had done and assured me it was time.

I scheduled the IVF appointment, and did my level best to quell the thoughts that chased me around at night. *But what happens if that doesn't work?* I put on my brave face and reminded myself there were other options; maybe a surrogate or perhaps adoption. I reminded myself of friends who had taken these routes, and they had become incredible parents. They had beautiful children who loved them no matter how they got here. I was a child who grew up in a nontraditional family; my aunt took me in as her own. It had worked out for the most part. So why couldn't I do that? And suddenly, just like that, this period of endless uncertainty gave way to a deep hope of possibility again. Like shaking the beach sand that had been kicked up in my face by the wind, I could suddenly begin to see things differently. I had to strip away the bullshit, be less afraid, and stop keeping score with myself. I had to stop thinking about what I wasn't and shift my mind to think about who I could become: an incredible mother, regardless of how the baby came to me.

September arrived, and I made the drive to a fertility clinic in Tysons Corner, about an hour away from where I lived in the city. We started with the preliminary IVF testing process, blood panels, pelvic ultrasound checks, and a tubal patency test, where they flush fluid through your fallopian tubes to ensure nothing is blocked. Also known as the longest thirty seconds of my life. All results were positive; there were no significant callouts. Part of me had hoped they would find something so I could get some answers, and we could fix whatever needed to be fixed. But there was nothing wrong that was clear. My next visit, which would start the IVF treatment process was scheduled for the last week of October. I wanted to reserve the week before for my birthday—I wanted to enjoy it at the beach with my husband.

As I arrived at the beach, I was expecting my period. That Saturday, I woke up—still nothing. I tried not to freak out and bust out a pregnancy test right away. I woke up Sunday, but there was still no period. I convinced myself to hold off until we got home, but I knew the signs by now. Coffee would start to taste weird; my boobs would be sore, I would always have this odd craving for cereal anytime throughout the day. The signs showed up, but I waited until Monday morning to test them. I woke up and grabbed one of the extra pregnancy tests I had lying around. The word pregnant showed up quickly on the test. But, I didn't get excited this time, nor did I rush to call the doctor's office. I had been here before. And that's the thing with pregnancy loss; it robs the joy or any excitement that one would typically have in this process. I knew too much about what could happen. So, I managed my emotions and went on about my day. No fanfare, no planning. Just rinse and repeat.

We made it to our twenty-week appointment at the beginning of February; it was the longest we had been pregnant. This appointment was the "big" one because it was the anatomy scan. Getting to this point felt like the longest-held breath I had ever taken. The sonographer, Pragati, was our regular—she had been with us throughout these last few years. By now, she was like family. She had been witness to my rawest moments. She knew what we had gone through, and we knew what to expect from her; she checked a few things internally with me first; we were all silent until she announced, "I will check on the baby."

She walked us through each body part and explained that the heartbeat looked excellent and robust, the hands and legs looked great, all parts of the heart looked good, and all blood flow was where it should be. As she showed us the parts on the screen and moved the transducer over my abdomen, my body grew tighter, and Brad held my hand. With each new body part, my grip became stronger.

Pragati smiled with her next announcement, "I am happy to tell you, you have a healthy, active baby girl." As soon as the words came out of her mouth, my whole body shuttered with relief on the table. Pragati handed me the images of our healthy baby girl and gave me a massive hug. And this time, we were escorted through the front lobby of the office. It was the first time I had nothing to hide. I walked out of the front lobby with my head up, a hand holding my healthy baby bump, and the other holding an ultrasound picture of my healthy baby girl.

It was a hot and humid Baltimore summer day in July; I drove to Towson, a suburb a few miles outside of the city when a message from Mary Ann, my therapist, popped up on my car's info screen, "I can't wait to meet her!"

I had done the drive to my therapist's office so many times by now, but this drive felt different. I had the windows cracked slightly to get that sweet summer air into my lungs as I took in intentional breaths of gratitude, joy, and peace. Most of my drives up were generally made in silence so I could get present and grounded before my session, even though I was rushing to get there on time from work. Today, though, I was taking my sweet time up the major highway. I pulled into the parking spot outside the building and looked into the rearview mirror. My sweet, healthy, beautiful baby girl was sleeping so peacefully in the car seat. I walked into Mary Ann's office and was greeted with a hug from her as we both shed happy tears.

"She's really here!" Mary Ann cooed marveling at me as she wrapped her hands around my arms, taking another look at my sleeping baby. We walked into her office and I sat on the couch, in the same spot where it had all begun, so many years earlier.

"Can you believe it, Jam? She's here!" I sniffed back more tears and laid a hand gently on her sleeping head.

"Remember that first appointment almost three years ago? You had your running shoes on with a skirt! All I could think was, 'this woman can't stop running! She is just running through life, and if she doesn't stop, she's seriously going to hurt herself!' But we have come a long way!" She motioned to my daughter, and my heart swelled with pride. We both smiled because we each knew she thought I was just going to get up in the middle of that first session and run right out the door. But I didn't. I leaned into the hard. She, along with so many others, had helped me stay brave. I could feel Mary Ann's pride, like a proud aunty, for overcoming all that I had been through. I had not given up, but, most importantly, I had stopped running.

I could never have imagined my journey to motherhood would be such a marathon. It was the most important race of my life because it taught me how to heal and accept, and ultimately prepared me to be a better mother today. I had to come down, to come up and go through this human experience to realize the kind of mother I wanted to show up as. I kept the losses along the way, and I always will hold them in my heart;

I thank them for showing me the path, and pushing me to run when I had to run, and rest when I had to rest. Without them, I wouldn't be the mother I am today.

Jami Crist is a mother, brand, community builder and connector of people, organizations, and communities. One of her greatest joys is helping businesses make more out of their marketing. She's a champion for women— challenging the status quo by living as her most authentic and radical self. She resides full-time in Baltimore, MD, and enjoys her summers at Rehoboth Beach, Delaware, with her family. Jami had a challenging journey in becoming a mother, experiencing four pregnancy losses, two in the second trimester, and three surgeries, all in less than two and a half years. There were no answers from the medical system on why these losses were happening, rendering Jami feeling so alone. Whenever she received the news that she would lose her baby or miscarry, she instantly began researching other women's stories— looking for others who had been through this horrific experience and, most importantly, search desperately for what they did to get through it. Did they get help? Did they get pregnant later? If so, how did they have a successful pregnancy? Finding such stories from women was hard, even though she scowered the internet. She would find a few posts on social media or a blog post here and there, but it was tough. She needed to look forward to getting her baby in her arms, healthy, safe, and sound. She realized she needed a book to guide her, a place where she could hear other women's stories, to be a guiding light in this dark journey. But she couldn't find one. This led her to creating her first anthology *The Losses We Keep: Fertility, Loss and Never-Ending Hope.* You can connect with Jami on Instagram @JamiCrist.

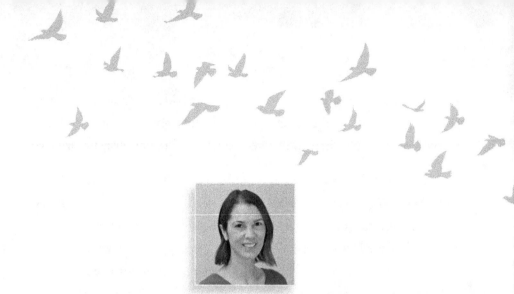

YOU'LL COME AROUND

Kyle Kassa

You are managing this so well.

You are so strong.

I do not know how you do it.

Awkwardly bent over a chair in a small office of the fertility clinic, I braced myself as the nurse, Emma, injected the thick neon yellow fluid into my right ass cheek.

"I am so sorry, Kyle. But you are tough, you will get through this," Emma assured me.

The sun, beaming down through the office window overlooking Baltimore's Inner Harbor, reflected rays of bright light off the water. Not a single cloud floated in the cyan sky. One might surmise that based on the view from this seventh-floor window, it was a warm spring day in the city. But those of us who had stepped outside that morning knew the temperature was the type of bone-chilling cold that shot needles through your spine when you braced yourself for the bitter February air.

As I massaged the area where the liquid was burning my butt muscle, Emma explained the precautions I would need to take after receiving this dose of methotrexate. "No alcohol, and be sure to wear extra coverage and SPF in the sun because you can burn very easily. As we discussed on the phone, you will have to wait at least three months before you can attempt another pregnancy, unfortunately. Try to enjoy your trip."

A few hours later, I crammed into a window seat on my rescheduled flight to Puerto Rico. Heading to a bachelorette party, one day late thanks to my emergency injection, I tried to imagine enjoying myself. Considering I could not have any alcohol and needed to avoid the sun at all costs, it did not seem promising. However, after managing to acquire THC gummies for the trip at the final hour, I was looking forward to being stoned for most of the time. Staring out at the clouds through the portal of the airplane window, I reflected on how different I was from the woman I had been just two years ago.

On another frigid February day, in a previous life, I was sitting in my car in the Target parking lot, peeling the aluminum seal off my brand-new prenatal vitamin bottle. It had only been an hour since I left my OB-GYN's office to have my IUD removed. I told them I wanted to get pregnant. They told me to start taking prenatals right away.

"Some women become pregnant very quickly after having their IUD removed," she said with a twinkle in her eye. "You'll want to ensure you're giving the baby essential vitamins and nutrients immediately!"

As I swallowed the recommended dosage of the berry-flavored chew, the butterflies flitting around my stomach were a true indicator of what I knew as they pulled the IUD out. I was ready to become a mother.

A jarring bump thrust me back into the present as our plane bounced along the tarmac. I texted my husband Sam from the San Juan airport: *Landed.* His response was brief: *Phew. Try to enjoy your trip, love you.*

My husband is a man of few words. When I met Sam eleven years prior, his lack of spoken words was mysterious and refreshing. As a twenty-two-year-old college student, I was already sick of conversations with men that consisted of blowing smoke up my ass. Sam was smart and funny, and his quiet confidence had made me feel safe for over a decade. Although I appreciated the safety, I wanted more emotion from him regarding our current situation. I wanted a page-long text saying how sorry he was that this was happening, that he was also feeling devastated, but we would get through it together. Instead of expressing my desolation and telling him what I needed, I continued to swallow my feelings down, past the baseball-sized lump that was continuing to grow in my throat, dropping down to fill my empty childless stomach.

The methotrexate Emma had syringed into my body was the result of our most recent IVF failure: a suspected ectopic pregnancy. This second attempt at an embryo transfer was preceded by a failed transfer the previous fall. A failed transfer is simple: the attempt to implant the embryo in my uterus did not work, resulting in a negative blood pregnancy test ten days post-transfer. The phone calls with results from the fertility clinic always came during the workday. On the day the doctor called to tell me the first transfer did not work, I glanced around my office to take inventory of how many people were there, as I tried to blink away the tears that were blurring my vision. *Didn't I already know this is what he would say?* The negative pregnancy test I had taken that morning was already collecting dust on our bathroom sink. But the doctor's confirmation of what I already knew felt cruel. All that work, all that time, all that waiting. And I still was not pregnant. Suddenly flooded with hopelessness, I could not wrap my head around why this was happening to us. Why didn't we deserve to have a child as easily as it felt like everyone else did?

I decided my body needed a break from IVF. It was fall, and the plan was to regroup and start another transfer prep in January. I attempted to recover mentally as well but only retreated further into myself. During the holiday season, pregnancy announcements on social media appeared every time I opened Instagram and Facebook. At the sight of each announcement, envy flooded my body with bitterness. Unfair thoughts about these couples occupied my mind as I measured their years of marriage compared to ours and decided it was not their turn, but ours. I had created a Pregnancy Competition in my head, and with each negative pregnancy test, I felt I was falling further behind, sure to come in last place or be disqualified.

Congratulations! I commented on their posts, all the while judging their good fortune, as if it were stealing from mine.

As we approached the second embryo transfer, I restricted my hope. Whenever a slice of yearning would try to splinter its way into my heart, I immediately shunned it. The universe would do whatever it wanted with me, regardless of my hopes. Thanks to COVID-19 regulations, I sat alone in the clinic for the second time, awaiting the procedure's start. Part of transfer prep is to arrive with a full bladder as this makes it easier for the doctor to see the uterus for embryo implantation. Upon arrival at the clinic, the woman at the front desk explained that my doctor was running behind schedule and the wait would be longer than expected. As my bladder continued to fill with the copious amounts of water I had consumed on the drive to the clinic, I tried desperately to distract myself from my physical discomfort. The waiting room was expansive with lofty ceilings and multiple televisions, always airing HGTV. Because all women must prioritize home improvement, of course. Unable to escape my expanding bladder pain with the newest episode of *Fixer Upper,* I found my gaze traveling to the other women in the waiting room, wondering what brought them to this moment. Were they here trying to have their first baby? Their second? Were they single women freezing their eggs to buy them more time on biology's ticking clock? The realization that we were all here to conquer some great fertility adversity comforted me like a warm blanket, straight from the dryer: I was not here alone.

In the procedure room, my full bladder made its unhappiness clear as I stared idly at the ceiling covered in glow-in-the-dark stars. Meant to provide a sense of weightlessness for women lying on the table awaiting implantation, the stars only made me yearn for the simplicity of childhood. If only I could time travel to my childhood bedroom and gaze up at these glowing galaxies while I giggled with girlfriends and ate pizza. I'd give anything to teleport back to that time when the biggest worry I had was whether I had enough time to take a quick swim in the river before my mom wanted me home for dinner; I craved that version of myself.

Ten days later, Emma had called to explain that, while my pregnancy test was positive, my pregnancy hormone, known as hCG, was much lower than they liked to see at this stage. Feigning shock at her news, I mentally recounted the past five days where I had obsessively taken pregnancy test after pregnancy test, comparing pink lines on the stick to the picture of the pink lines on my phone from the previous day's result. *Were today's lines darker? They were supposed to darken each day, right?* Mine seemed to stay the same. I compared my photos to those in online forums where other women sought answers that no one could provide.

"What does that mean?" I asked Emma.

"It could mean that the embryo implanted later than we expected, and you are pregnant but just not as far along. We will need you to repeat blood work in two days. If the hCG doubles, then we are clear—for now."

For now.

"What if it doesn't double?"

"Let's just wait and see."

Over the course of one week and daily blood work, my hCG continued to rise, but it never doubled. During this time, hopeful family members and friends would frequently check in for important updates. While well-meaning, the check-ins pressured me to provide news to others when I had not had time to process the information for myself.

Eventually, Emma expressed the team's concerns that I was experiencing an ectopic pregnancy. As a technician performed an ultrasound to locate the embryo, I watched the screen and desperately searched her face for a sign of recognition that she had found what she was looking for. But all I could see was confusion. They could not track down the embryo but knew it was somewhere inside my body due to the slightly rising hCG levels. Crippling fear consumed me. The idea that there was something lost somewhere inside of me dominated my every thought, and I wanted nothing more than to escape my body. *How could I have followed all the rules and still ended up here?*

It was late when I arrived in San Juan, and my girlfriends were already out when I turned up at the house. While changing into my clubbing outfit, I decided to dig into my THC gummies. Although I was an avid stoner in college, I had only been high one other time in the past five years during a trip to Breckenridge (when in Rome!). After swallowing half of the pineapple-infused chew, I figured I might as well eat the whole thing. Heading out the door to meet my friends, I checked my phone. There was a text from a friend who had suggested this type of THC for the trip: *I forgot to mention, you should only take a quarter or half of those gummies since it has been so long for you.*

Whoops.

Thirty minutes later, a fit of giggles engulfed me, temporarily relieving me of my sorrow. Dripping with sweat, I found a release while dancing with my friends. I surrendered to the music, warm air, and great company to provide the solace I so desperately craved. After spending so much time waiting for the other shoe to drop and preparing for unwelcome news, I almost forgot what it was like to live in the present and feel this good.

In my twenties, I was not sure I ever wanted children. My father was an alcoholic who died from an accidental overdose when I was twenty-eight. Addiction and mental health struggles plagued both sides of my family for generations, and I worried about passing these issues on to my children. When discussing these concerns with Sam, he simply said, "You'll come around." How annoying when he turned out to be right. Something changed in my thirties, as I observed friends and family members become parents. Witnessing my beloved niece grow into a capable, intelligent, and kind-hearted human and watching her play sports gave me immense joy. Suddenly, I yearned to feel this happiness watching my own children. I explained my change of heart to Sam, and we decided to "pull the goalie" and have tons of fun, unprotected sex. Once the doctor removed my IUD, we figured we would be pregnant by summer. Eleven long months later, I found myself staring down at a positive pregnancy test on our bathroom counter.

On a crisp, sunny Saturday, about one year after having my IUD taken out, I woke up feeling hopeful and happy. It was the best kind of Saturday: a Saturday with zero plans. Scheduled to see my OB-GYN the following Monday for our inaugural ultrasound, Sam and I were excited to see the baby's heartbeat for the first time. After shopping in the morning, we decided to meet up with friends for lunch. I popped into the bathroom at the restaurant for a pee break, and my heart sank as I was flushing the toilet. There was blood.

An intense wave of claustrophobia set in as the walls of the bathroom stall closed in around me and escape felt unobtainable. Although bleeding is common in early pregnancy, I instantly understood this was not regular pregnancy bleeding. Rushing back to our table, I whispered to Sam that we needed to leave. We quickly explained to our friends that I was pregnant, was bleeding, and needed to go. For the first time, I experienced the feeling of having that exciting moment of sharing my pregnancy news with loved ones ripped from me.

Once we reached the car, I called my OB-GYN's emergency weekend phone line. The nurse on the line explained with a calm and straightforward voice that it could be regular pregnancy bleeding but could be a miscarriage. I could go to the ER if I started filling up a pad with blood in an hour or less, but there would be nothing they could do if I were miscarrying, and it might be better to stay home where I could be more comfortable.

As I lay in the fetal position, consumed by physical pain, I could feel Sam's helplessness radiating across the room. We stared aimlessly into the blue light of the television screen, wishing it could break us free from reality. Despair swallowed me whole. I wanted someone, anyone, to save me from the pain and heartbreak I knew was coming.

The day I hoped to hear my baby's heartbeat for the first time, my doctor confirmed I had experienced a miscarriage and no fetal tissue remained in my uterus. There would be no heartbeat. Sitting in the leather chair opposite his desk, I stared blankly past my doctor's shoulder, out to the parking lot where Sam sat waiting in the car. Swallowing bile that was creeping up my throat, I suddenly became conscious of the young resident in a white coat who was standing uncomfortably in the corner of the room, observing. *This is the last place on earth this man wants to be right now*, I thought sadly. *Me too, Doc.*

We began testing with the fertility clinic in the summer. These tests were invasive, with their endless poking and prodding. I was beginning to have the sense that my body no longer belonged to me. It was like I was completely disconnecting from it to survive. After about a month of testing for both of us, Sam and I met with our doctor to review the results and discuss a treatment plan. *Why was this so hard for us?* we asked. *Where were we failing?*

"Unexplained infertility," the doctor announced, as he perused our file and then closed the pages as if the whole thing were open and shut.

What? While relieved to know we did not have the barriers that other couples with infertility face, it was hard to reconcile that there was simply no explanation for our struggle to get and stay pregnant. The doctor explained, approximately 40 percent of couples who have trouble conceiving fall under the diagnosis of unexplained infertility. While this number was comforting in a sense, it was frustrating that so many people experience this pain, and there are no clear answers as to why. Sifting through our options, we decided to pursue IVF as a way forward. I was ready to tackle this "project," taking diligent notes and preparing to approach IVF with the same tenacity I harbored when working on a school project or work deadline. It didn't take long for me to realize no one can quickly ace IVF.

While anticipating the injections, medications, and hormones would be the worst part of IVF, I was surprised to find the time commitment and uncertainty most taxing. I remained steadfast in my attempts to prove to myself that I could be the best wife, daughter, sister, friend, and employee, all while undergoing intensive fertility treatment, which involved daily 7:00 a.m. blood draws, transvaginal ultrasounds, mixing medications, and ensuring I followed the injection schedule precisely. And then there was the waiting. Waiting, waiting, waiting. Waiting for results that would dictate the treatment for the following day. Waiting for answers about when and if the egg retrieval would ever happen. My phone stayed glued to my hand all day at work while my heart skipped a beat with every vibration it emanated. More than once I wondered if any of this would be worth it.

After the miscarriage, I shared my experience on social media. Understanding that pregnancy held a one in four chance of loss, desperation to hear from others who had been through something similar compelled me to speak out about my experience. The response was astounding. Friends and acquaintances from high school, college, and beyond shared their experiences and described the deep loneliness and heartache I felt. Women I hardly even knew, opened up, some for the first time, that they had not shared their losses with anyone other than their partners due to the fear they would be judged or blamed for what happened to them. This fear of judgment had plagued me as well. As our infertility journey pressed on, I continued to share the IVF experience and losses on my social media. I was comforted by stories and similar emotions surrounding loss and infertility. Still, I could not help feeling resentful about other comments on my post and frequently daydreamed about how I wanted to respond to them.

You are so strong. No, I am not! I am resorting to posting about this on social media because I am deeply suffering and hoping someone can explain how to survive this!

You are managing this so well. I am drowning, I am heartbroken, I am LONELY. Please someone tell me this will all work out for the best.

I do not know how you do it. I don't either. But, I don't have a choice.

While it appeared to everyone else that I was being open and honest about my journey, I was not expressing my true feelings to those I loved. While donning a mask that portrayed a woman of strength and resilience, anger and resentment had been curdling inside of me like expired milk since the miscarriage. It didn't help that people tiptoed around me because they didn't know what to say. At parties and gatherings, pity was radiating off of every surface. In my attempt to seek relief from my loneliness by sharing my story so publicly, I had unwittingly created new resentments caused by the intrusive stares. In an effort to connect as an act of survival, I had sacrificed the intimacy with myself that I had spent a lifetime creating. My body was not solely mine anymore but had been offered up to science so that it could bring forth a baby. The experiences I had hoped I would have in this process had been snatched away by grief and time. There was no time to process, but rather, I went from obsessively googling to worrying, to wondering, to fearing, silently begging someone, anyone, to tell me it was all going to be okay. It would take me months, if not years, to unravel the complicated feelings I couldn't identify in real time. It felt as if I had nothing for myself anymore, not my body, not my experiences, not my feelings.

I went to the bachelorette party with a miscarriage, one failed embryo transfer, and one ectopic pregnancy under my belt, and when I got home, the methotrexate forced me to pause fertility treatment for at least three months due to toxicity levels in my body. While Sam remained optimistic that we would eventually have a child, I was becoming convinced our future as parents was nonexistent. Fear of the unknown and unkind thoughts toward myself burdened my brain and prevented me from experiencing the joy happening in my present life. I was consumed by resentment toward my body for not doing what I had always been taught a woman's body was made to do. Hadn't it been shoved down our throats since middle school that not using protection during sex would result in pregnancy every single time? There must have been something wrong with me. I must have deserved this in some way, and my inability to grow my own biological family had been some type of atonement for past behavior. The negative and toxic thoughts raged on, so rather than experiencing my life as it was happening to me, I found myself searching for every type of distraction known to womankind, desperate to avoid my thoughts and fears. I spent every waking moment listening to audiobooks or watching television. The Real Housewives of Potomac, Salt Lake City, and Orange County became my new best friends. Nothing will make a person feel more normal than watching rich women scream at each other over the dinner table whilst wielding butter knives as potential weapons.

Sam and I had decided to wait until the end of summer to attempt another embryo transfer. We arrived at the clinic early on a warm September morning. On the drive, I gazed out the window at the cars zooming by us on the highway, forcing positive thoughts into my mind.

Today is different from the other days, even if they feel the same.

You could get pregnant today.

The baby could live.

You could have the life of which you have dreamed.

For the first time, Sam was able to attend the transfer procedure with me since COVID restrictions had been lifted in the clinic. Together, we sat under the glow-in-the-dark galaxy with a nurse and my doctor, waiting for the embryologist to bring in our embryo and confirm our identities.

"Ready?" the doctor asked.

I scooched my butt all the way to the edge of the cold table, the thin protective paper underneath me crinkling loudly. I clenched Sam's hand as we watched the ultrasound screen above our heads showing the embryo implanting into my uterus. In addition to the bladder reaching maximum capacity during an embryo transfer, another piece of intimacy was lost in the process. After the embryo was released from the catheter inserted inside my vagina, the doctor removed the tube and handed it to the embryologist to confirm the embryo had been released from the catheter. As the embryologist checked on this, I had to continue lying on my back with the doctor and nurse stationed at the end of the table. While many lucky couples become pregnant in the privacy of their bedrooms by participating in what I hope is pleasurable sex, Sam and I were trying to get pregnant, legs splayed apart like a Thanksgiving turkey, while making small talk about the weather with my seventy-something-year-old male doctor. I would have gone to the ends of the Earth and back to have a child with this man I loved dearly, so I put on my best smile and told the doctor how excited I was for changing leaves and sweater weather.

The ten-day waiting period between transfer day and pregnancy test day was a fresh version of hell. The seconds felt like hours, and the clock on my phone taunted me, as it leered back at my stares, refusing to move forward. It makes sense that during this time I needed to behave like a pregnant person. While some doctors are okay with caffeine intake, my doctor advised that I avoid caffeine and high-intensity exercise, in addition to all the usual restrictions placed upon pregnant women. After my miscarriage and first two failed IVF transfers, I found this part to be the cruelest. In all three instances, my mind had convinced my body that I was pregnant. While ten days does not typically feel particularly long, it had been enough time for me to become attached to the idea that my body was carrying another human, and finding out this wasn't true had carried an extra layer of devastation in those experiences. I dreaded having this happen again but I knew that up until this point, I had done everything in my power to become pregnant and would just need to wait and see. If anything, IVF and infertility were teaching me that no matter how hard we try or how much we yearn for it, we can not control time.

"You're pregnant!" Emma chirped over the line when I answered my phone on the day of my pregnancy test, the relief in her voice palpable. While joy and excitement peeked out from the shadows with the news, uneasiness pulled the curtain shut on any hope that was headed our way.

To my utter disappointment, a healthy pregnancy did not cure my fear or the trauma that had been induced by my miscarriage. Fear sank into my bones, and it was difficult for me to accept that I would ever be able to carry a healthy baby to term. Bitterness and envy still reared their ugly heads when realizing I would not have traditional pregnancy experiences. Because I had been so open about my journey with friends and family, they all knew right away when I was pregnant. There would be no cutesy presentations to our moms with surprise ultrasound photos and cards slyly stating, "Congrats, Grandma!" Never mind the countless restless nights when I woke up drenched in sweat, my heart racing at the speed of light and feeling like it might explode right from my chest onto the bed—*something bad is going to happen.*

During my first trimester, Sam and I experienced some marriage issues that resulted in both of us becoming more curious about our relationship and ourselves. Deciding to dig deep into self-reflection, I began learning more about myself as a human. I knew I needed to heal from a significant amount of trauma from my childhood and the years of loss and fertility battles. It was vital for me to determine the types of coping mechanisms that could propel me into a solid foundation for motherhood.

As a child of an alcoholic, it became second nature for me to hide my feelings and needs. Never wanting to burden others with my childish trials and tribulations became integral to my personality, shaping me into a people pleaser to my core. I could not fathom the notion of expressing my emotional needs but was quick to absorb the needs and wants of everyone around me. Even when I would share my difficulties in life, such as my infertility struggles on social media, my words were hollow, or I would make a joke to cover up my pain. Hiding behind a mask of bravery and resilience, the only person I was hurting by not telling anyone how deep my wounds had become was myself.

With this pregnancy, I talked to people. Not on social media, but to their faces and in writing. When family members and friends would ask the age-old question directed at pregnant women, "How are you feeling?" I would answer honestly:

"I am scared this baby will not survive."

"I am terrified to be excited."

"I am worried about the person I will become if I experience another loss."

I kept details of this pregnancy close to my heart, sharing minimally on social media this time around. But one day, at a friend's birthday party, an acquaintance pulled me aside to express gratitude for the IVF videos I had posted.

"I keep going back to watch your videos. They make me feel less alone, thank you," she admitted quietly.

It reminded me of myself during the ectopic pregnancy, frantically searching for comparable stories on Google only to come up short.

Conversations like these gave me the sense that the universe had been looking out for me all along, and the loss and devastation I experienced could help other women navigate the muddy waters of infertility. But I needed to balance holding space for others while not giving too much of myself away.

One day in February, three years after having my IUD removed, I lay on the couch on my back with my hands placed on my stomach. I watched as little ripples thumped the surface of my belly and felt butterfly-like twitches inside me. Sitting still at that moment, feeling my baby girl moving inside me, cemented me to the Earth and provided me with an overwhelming sense of calm. There were still days when none of it felt real, and I couldn't believe I had made it to the third trimester of pregnancy. I still glanced down at the toilet paper every time I peed to check for blood. My heart rate still skyrocketed at every doctor's appointment and ultrasound, convinced this would be the day someone would have to break the news to me that something had gone wrong and I wouldn't get to meet this baby after all. During one appointment, as I stared at the sonographer's face, searching for signs that my baby was okay, a wide grin came over his face. "Whoa! That's a very active baby!" he chuckled aloud. The hope, intimacy, mindfulness, and self-love that had deteriorated over the past three years began to grow along with the life inside of me—albeit slowly. As I pressed my hand onto my belly, an elbow or a foot pressed back, reminding me that worrying about something bad happening would not stop it from happening.

Today, this moment was exceptional, and that was enough. Laying in the same spot where I had writhed in physical and emotional agony two years before during the miscarriage, I felt this baby telling me, *I am here.* It was as if we were promising each other that no matter the outcome of the pregnancy or the future, we would have these moments together and nothing could take them away. It was enough, in this fleeting moment in time, for me to know we were safe and happy.

Kyle Kassa is a proud millennial who loves to read, watch movies, pet dogs, exercise, and try to make people laugh. She has a master's degree in rehabilitation counseling from Michigan State University (Go Green!) and has devoted her life and career to helping others. She currently works at the Community College of Baltimore County, where she serves underprivileged students in workforce development. Kyle is excited to have this opportunity to share her infertility journey with you and hopes it can provide hope and comfort for everyone who reads it. She lives in Baltimore, Maryland with her husband, their magical daughter, and their two senior citizen dogs. You can connect with Kyle on Instagram @kylekassa19.

DEEP BREATH IN, SLOW BREATH OUT

Kate Rowe

"If you don't get your shit together, you're going to miss the birth of your baby."

That's not exactly what she said, but in that moment, that's what I heard as the nurse explained to me they would automatically put me under for twenty-four hours if I passed out. Laid out and twisted onto the cesarean table, waiting for them to open me up, all I could do was hope.

It had been a long few days in the Labor and Delivery COVID-19 suite. On Monday, I had narrowly escaped a we-might-be-having-a-baby-today checkup because of elevated blood pressure. I had symptoms of preeclampsia, a common but serious condition in pregnant women. Still, I wasn't ready to pop out a baby at thirty-six weeks, alone, while my husband was sick with the virus we had carefully avoided for years, until the time for our child to be born. Two days later, clad in my softest bamboo pregnancy pajamas, I recorded yet another high blood pressure reading, plus a positive COVID test; I reluctantly admitted it was time to go and get this baby out. It felt strange to be grateful for sickness, but because we were both testing positive, my husband Tom could join me in Labor and Delivery; I didn't know it then, but that would be one of the greatest gifts I've ever received.

Five days later, I was relegated to my side, riding a peanut-shaped birthing ball, coughing up what felt like an entire lung while two masked doctors checked my dilation; it didn't feel like such a gift then. But this wasn't my first hospital rodeo.

Six years earlier, after enduring years of misdiagnosing severe abdominal pains as "stress" (cue the eye roll) and IBS, a scan revealed a cancerous granulosa cell tumor—a type of ovarian cancer—over my left ovary. My incredible oncology team worked quickly to perform a laparoscopic oophorectomy, a minimally invasive surgery to remove the tumor, as well as my ovary and tube on that side. Looking back, that first recovery felt like nothing. On paper, I know I had major surgery, but the memory resonates more like a sour stomach on vacation—days off from work, minimal scarring, coloring books, movies, and naps with the dog. My biggest hurdle was wanting to rush back to my life. I was in my twenties and felt like I was missing out, like everything was happening without me, and I was less of a person for not being there.

Once I had recovered and returned to "normal life," it only took a few months to realize my diagnosis had opened up a new path forward for me. A cancer diagnosis, followed by surgery that had removed my ovary, had shifted something in my heart. I knew this when I returned to work and found myself behind a closed office door, lying on the floor having an out-of-body experience. The world was moving at triple speed, and I saw a timelapse of people shuffling through life, blurred and busy. *Was this what I have survived for? What had I rushed my healing for?* I had proof that life was short, and I realized in that moment, I was ready for change. So, I made some decisions that included saying a bittersweet farewell to my nine-to-five and starting a small business with my friend to help promote other local small businesses. My husband and I went to couple's therapy, and we started planning for the future. The path I had been put on was mine to blaze and it was extraordinary!

We'd been planning a family trip to Sweden; my entire family was excited to visit places we hadn't been to since I was a teenager. I loved the idea of sharing our ancestral culture with Tom. As I looked out the window of our hotel room, I was in awe of the beauty and charm of Stockholm. I checked the time and saw I had a few minutes to spare before meeting the rest of the crew for dinner, so I popped into my email as one often automatically does in downtime—swiping away junk into my trash and flagging things that would need attention for later. I pulled up an alert from my oncologist. I had gone in for my routine six-month check-up right before our trip, happy to have graduated from going in every three months to six months for blood work. I opened the patient portal, fully expecting to read that my levels were unremarkable, when three words caught my attention: Abnormal Mass Detected. *WTF!?* After quickly and quietly talking myself off a ledge of panic, I reminded myself that I'm not a doctor, and it would be wise not to speculate on what that meant without context. There was no use in alarming my family when I had no clarity, especially in a foreign country.

I tried to swallow the words along with the wine that night. But the dam could only hold so long and by 3:00 a.m. I woke up, drowning. The room was still, but my mind was swirling with thoughts, feelings, and questions . . . *What did this mean? Another surgery? Would I need a full hysterectomy? Would I never be able to have kids? Was I dying? Was I going to be sick for the rest of my life? What if I could never be a mom?* I tried to lay undisturbed, calm myself down, and will away the panic that was building up inside me. Hot and cold waves of fear and anxiety flushed through my body as I woke up my husband. A full nightmare was starting to come into focus, and the floor fell out from under me. Tears soaked through my shirt. He held me as I shook and gasped for air. My body, tense and aching, was hollowed out from a loss, before it even happened. At that moment, my first fertility panic attack opened up a cage of questions that led to an infinite unknown.

Just one day after I received the news that they had found an abnormal mass, we flew home as regularly scheduled, and I immediately contacted my doctor. She confirmed the mass was another cancerous tumor growing on my right ovary. She made it clear it was not a recurrence but another tumor. *Lucky me*, I thought as she delivered the news over the phone. Her recommendation was immediate surgical removal. As I quickly considered what was to happen next, all I could think about was how I wanted to be a mom—and that I wanted to carry my baby in my own body. I expressed this desire, and she assured me that, as a mother herself, she understood. Together, we decided another oophorectomy to remove my remaining ovary and tube could be done without removing my uterus.

I had one month to assemble a team that I could discuss the possibilities with, and quickly my days were filled with appointments with fertility teams where IVF was confirmed as risky but our best, perhaps only, route forward. We would have one chance to go through the treatments to stimulate egg production—one last hurrah for my only remaining ovary before they removed it, along with the cancer. IVF days are not easy; it's a forced hormone roller coaster that leaves you battered and bruised from daily injections and weekly clinic visits, the daily shots, balloon tests, and physical exams were grueling. There were days it all felt too heavy, but I knew I couldn't stop. This was our only shot.

My egg retrieval was on a Tuesday and my oophorectomy was scheduled for exactly two weeks later. It seemed they needed just a few days for my insides to recover before I went under the knife again. Thankfully, the retrieval was a success, and I could at least rest my mind a little, knowing we had embryos frozen for the future. I realized that short-lived rest still counts.

Dressed in my hospital best, which included blue sticky extra extra large socks and a thin '80s print gown that opened in the back, I was connected to all the tubes and scanners in prep for surgery. I've always been curious when it comes to medical procedures, and, despite the severity of the situation, I focused on chatting with the technicians and asked if I could stay awake to watch the surgery on the big monitor while they counted me down from ten . . . nine . . . eight . . . seven . . . I blinked my eyes open and realized it was dark outside. Surgery had been scheduled for the morning, so my head was spinning to see I had lost an entire day. *What happened? What day was it? Where was I?* Tom was right there by my side and squeezed my hand, reassuring me that after almost seven hours, while the surgery had been complicated it had been successful.

As the events were explained to me later, "messy" was the descriptor that stood out the most. This tumor had not been as compact as the previous one and could have been further impacted by the IVF injections, making it more difficult to remove fully. They attempted a laparoscopic surgery but had to pivot and make a much larger incision. I looked down at the bandages covering my belly, tucked into my giant gauze underwear. Laying in the hospital bed, I could already tell this was a far cry from the first surgery. The room filled with flowers and friends and we laughed about gas—how I was so desperate to pass it after surgery, but not so much that I might rip my stitches. I went home to recover in bed with our dog, who had conveniently decided it was the perfect time to tear her other ACL so that she could lay in bed with me.

My oncologist recommended we wait at least a year before even thinking about pregnancy. She promised to discuss it with her colleagues, and I promised to spend time recovering. But this time around took so much more out of me, in every sense of the word. It wasn't just a physical recovery, but a mental and emotional one too. This surgery had rocked my body, and I had stitches that stretched from my belly button to my underwear line to prove it. It was nearly impossible for me to do anything other than lie in bed with my dog and my thoughts. This wasn't just a tumor they cut out of me, but part of my womanhood; part of my body, my worth, my being. This critically important piece of my body, that I had taken for granted all my life was now gone. Did that mean I was less of a woman than I had been before? Suddenly, everytime I looked in the mirror, I didn't know who I even was. As I took in the reflection of this woman who had survived cancer, not once, but twice, I felt a profound loss of identity. People kept telling me I was brave, but I just felt something akin to disoriented. My priorities changed; all of a sudden I no longer cared about work deadlines, but became dedicated to physical therapy. Yet again, my path was shifting. I was coming to understand that some scars don't just alter your body, but your entire self.

Once I had healed enough to do things independently, I felt the urge to find something, a hobby, to help me get active. I wanted some sort of stimulation, but I knew I had my limits. No more HIIT workouts for me, but sitting around coloring in my adult coloring book wasn't exactly cutting it either. So, I tried yin yoga and meditation. I learned how to play "Take Me Home, Country Roads" on the guitar. I tried watercolors and painted adorable pictures of dogs. Then, a friend invited me to a pottery class. I had thrown on the pottery wheel from a young age through college, so my interest was piqued. We laughed as we played in the mud, and I welcomed the escape from my current mental space. I made a small cup, and when I went back to glaze it, I scheduled another class. I've always been quick to recognize energy levels, and when talking to the owner and teachers, I knew almost instantly that I wanted to be part of this community. I enrolled in a six-week class. Then another. And another. My skills started to return and grow, and they asked me to join the team. Then, I sold a mug, and then, I sold a bowl. I sold another mug (to someone not related to me). Soon, what started as a way to recover from surgery transformed into the next chapter of my life.

Just after this beautiful, therapeutic, creative outlet turned to a new life path, the pandemic knocked us all off kilter. The studio closed temporarily, and we were all trapped inside our homes. I was scared for a whole new reason. Days were a stew of emotions: boredom, fear, annoyance, helplessness, freedom. Being forced to slow down and break away from the outside world pushed me in the direction of some big feelings and realizations. I reflected that my whole life, I had been rushing, forcing, hustling, frantically trying to climb higher, further, faster so I didn't miss out. *Miss out on what?* Call it "girlbossing" or "eldest daughter syndrome" or what it really was, *people-pleasing,* I could now see this behavior not as something I was, but something I did. And if this was an action, something I could choose to do, I could also choose to grow and change. I moved a pottery wheel into our rowhouse basement and decided to retreat into myself. I enjoyed the quiet time, the spinning wheel, and muddy hands.

I did my best to wait, and precisely one year later, I peppered my oncologist with questions about becoming pregnant. She had done her due diligence and taken my story to a tumor conference (which is a thing, apparently) and ultimately, after many conversations with colleagues, had come away with no clear answer. There was no history or precedence of someone in my situation. I was young-ish. I had no ovaries, but I did have a working uterus. And, although my type of tumor had fed off estrogen, there were no studies to determine if anything would or wouldn't happen. The oncology, fertility, and maternal-fetal medicine teams told us the choice was up to me. And that was easy.

I started IVF treatments immediately. My husband and I got into the routine of left cheek, right cheek, left cheek, right cheek; *Wait—didn't we just do this one?* Hot tip: a paper calendar is helpful to confirm which side you did the previous day. Masked up, squeezing each other's hands, we met with my fertility doctor regularly and were excited when implant day arrived. During the procedure, they talked me through what they were doing, including when the nurse left the room to check the tube under a scope. The embryo was so tiny they had to hold it under a microscope, before and after, to ensure it wasn't stuck on the side of the tube. It felt like we were in our own little sitcom, and the embryo was the star of the show. Seeing a nurse pop up in the drive-through style window of the exam room to report "It's out of here!" still makes me giggle!

There was no giggling during the excruciating ten days we had to wait before we could take a pregnancy test. But by then, I had waited over a year for this, so what was another ten days? The torturous waiting was forgotten the moment we saw the positive sign in bright pink. It was true and heartwarming JOY! The following days and weeks were a mix of happiness and relief. I took as many deep breaths and belly laughs as I could with the new stresses of being pregnant. As if one huge life shift wasn't enough, we were also in the middle of selling our house. I wasn't supposed to lift heavy boxes because I carried something more important.

Something about the moon kept me enchanted during this time, and I started internally calling the little thing growing inside me Luna. We had no idea what gender this little dot was, but everything inside me felt it was a girl. We'd drive to appointments, listen to '90s pop music in the waiting room, do the scan, and go home. Soon, the little dot on the ultrasound became a bigger dot. The bigger dot started blinking with a heartbeat. Our little miracle child was in there, and I was confident and comfortable that all I had been through was going to be worth it.

One morning Tom couldn't make a checkup so I sat alone in the exam room, waiting for the doctor to check in. She did the normal chatting, checkup, and scan, then left the room and came back a few minutes later. She explained she needed to do another scan, but she wasn't as chatty this time. Any ultrasound is frustrating when the tech won't tell you what they're seeing—it's just shades of gray to the untrained eye—but when a doctor won't speak, it shifts from annoying to alarming very quickly. She kept looking at the screen, then turned to look me deep in the eyes. And with one "I'm so sorry" my little Luna was gone. The tiny flicker of light inside me had burned out, and I just sat on the table unmovable and in shock. So fast. So permanent. So devastating. Pure and instant heartbreak. And then I had to call Tom. We cried on the phone until I had to hang up and sit alone in the exam room, waiting for my next steps. The supportive, reassuring staff probably walked me through what would happen next, and I can imagine I took notes, but I couldn't digest anything past "no heartbeat." I'll never know how I walked out of the office and drove myself home. I had been blinded by the fuzzy, warm light of a first pregnancy, and in an instant, someone sliced through the filter, and the fraying edges were precise. I could see all too clearly the cracks in the paint, water stains on the ceiling, and trash in the gutter. A new kind of numbness settled over me, and that night, we had a moonless night sky that was gray and heavy.

Without ovaries, I no longer had periods to complete the miscarriage, so I required a D&C procedure to remove the fetal tissue. Walking around in everyday life with a loss is indescribable. After the procedure, we had to wait for my numbers and body to recover before trying to get pregnant again. All I could do to move forward was think about moving forward; however, at an appointment almost a month later, my numbers still weren't in a good enough range. After more tests, the team confirmed there was debris in my uterus, causing my body to think I was still pregnant, and it would require yet another D&C. My belly churned with anger and heartbreak all over again, and I celebrated my thirty-sixth birthday on the operating table, having the remainder of my first pregnancy cleared out of me.

Our second round of IVF began that following summer, and once again, needles and paper calendars took over the bathroom counter in our one-bedroom apartment. We chose embryo number two and had a successful transfer in June. I remember watching a butterfly resting on the plants outside our bedroom window that day, hoping it was a little symbol of good luck as we moved toward this new beginning. We went through the motions and were always on high alert. The loss had sobered me and kept my optimism in check, ensuring I didn't feel too joyful about what this could mean; I knew now nothing was guaranteed. Ten days passed, and I was pregnant. The dot got bigger. The dot started blinking. I held my breath at our six-week appointment and let out a heavy sigh I'd probably been holding since June when we saw the first flicker. Six weeks grew into ten. Then the weeks became months, and soon, we were passed from fertility to the maternal-fetal medicine team. To them, I was just another high-risk case. Not rudely or dismissively, but in a regular this-is-our-job kind of way. I was so used to being coddled, first for my cancer, then for my IVF, then for my loss. It was jarring but strangely calming to have our doctor checkups become five-minute "keep doing what you're doing" sessions. The only thing that was out of the ordinary was that I could not lie entirely on my back. At every ultrasound, I had to lay on my side, or I'd start to get dizzy. The positioning proved difficult for the techs to get the images they needed, so I often had to return for additional scans. The working theory was that the baby was pressing on a blood vessel, which was annoying but not scary, and the doctor was confident we were both healthy, so we just kept doing what we were doing.

I truly loved being pregnant and still miss it often. It was weird and amazing and scary and life-affirming. And, although I never entirely gave in to the feeling, I felt good in my pregnant body. In the beginning, I found the foods I could eat without feeling nauseous—my favorite was a peanut butter and jelly sandwich using two frozen waffles. I gave in to my exhaustion until it turned to energy in the second trimester. I continued my acupuncture treatments and added an equally helpful and supportive chiropractor specializing in pregnancy as well as prenatal massages. I'm proud to say the training I gave my husband and coworkers to sense when I needed snacks is respected today.

The flickering dot grew to the size of a blueberry, a croissant, an action figure (Tom's favorite), and then . . . a baby boy. Throughout the days and weeks that would eventually turn into months, I would often see butterflies and almost always let out a little sigh when I did. Their gentle, colorful wings always eased my shoulders, echoing the hope from our implant day.

Appointments became more frequent, and baby prep had begun. I allowed myself to buy my first baby outfit with my best friend, a surprisingly poignant milestone I didn't realize I'd been holding back on. We ordered a crib that would fit in our apartment walk-in closet because, like so many, we still had not found a house in the insane market. My friends set up a mini baby shower, knowing I didn't want anything big. At the time, I focused on my very valid reason: we were still in a pandemic, and I was at high risk, especially as I was carrying around a plump watermelon. But, looking back, I know it was also my limiting unease that kept me from celebrating more. Of course, there's no going back, but I wish I could have let myself feel more of the true joy. The glimpses were there—the little ripples of hands and feet moving across my belly, and singing in the car on the way to work; it was just me and my little buddy, and I loved it. But every time I felt that love, the hot breath of fear hovered on the back of my neck.

And just a few weeks after the shower, Tom got COVID. This further proved to me that anything that can happen will. We tried to isolate ourselves in our apartment as best as possible, and I went to my appointment that Monday alone. At thirty-six weeks, they were taking no chances when my blood pressure tested high, and they sent me upstairs to Labor and Delivery. A slew of nurses and doctors came to check on me, giving me time in between to see if I would "calm down"— as if threatening me with childbirth weeks ahead of my due date, when I carried nothing but my wallet, keys, and phone with me, was the recipe for lowering blood pressure. After hours of monitoring, I shuffled out of that room by the skin of my teeth. I was prescribed morning and evening blood pressure checks and promised to call if I went above their noted levels. By Wednesday morning, I had surpassed the levels and had two positive rapid COVID tests. A call was made, and our bags were packed. That afternoon, we were directed to a particular hospital entrance, and Tom asked the fully covered nurse if he should bring in our bags from the car, and she said, without hesitation, "Absolutely. This is happening." If I had known I wouldn't breathe outside air again for ten days, I would have taken a few more deep cleansing breaths— and packed a few more snacks.

We began our journey in the Labor and Delivery COVID-19 suite, with its own circulating air cycle and a clean room separating us from the hallway. Every person who entered our room had to follow COVID protocols for covering up with masks, face shields, gowns, and gloves. It felt like we were living in a fish bowl with a city view, and much to my dismay, I was reunited with all my favorite tubes and monitors, plus new ones. I still couldn't lay on my back without the threat of passing out, and was alternating sides between doctor visits, which made my blood pressure cuff and primary IV attachments precarious and tangled. The beeps, blips, printouts, and pumps rang in my ears at all hours. Tom's chair folded out to a bed, if you could call it that, and we both coughed through the days and nights. The window that gave us a glimpse of the outside world quickly became littered with hospital cups of melted ice, charger cords, and chapstick. No one was allowed to visit, and we weren't going anywhere, but we were grateful when they allowed us to get a delivery of outside food, blankets, and pillows. Hot tip: always, *always* pack your pillow.

The team's confidence in being able to induce this birth was thwarted left and right by my baby's comfort inside the womb. We tried at dawn. We tried at midnight. Every shift lead had a new idea, and we tried them all. Meanwhile, I was lying on my side, slowly losing my mind. We were admitted on Wednesday afternoon, and by Friday night, I had started to feel trapped. I was tied to my bed by my IV, blood pressure cuff, and catheter; then, they added pneumatic compression sleeves on my legs. These inflatable sleeves wrapped around my calves and intermittently inflated to prevent blood from clotting in my legs. At the same time, my medications changed. As I lay there waiting for sleep to claim me, I could not ignore the grinding gears inflating the sleeves on my legs, gnawing away at my sanity as I could feel the medication flowing into my IV and through my blood. My skin was crawling, and I realized I was having a second panic attack. At some point during the night, a doctor shook me awake, notifying me that my oxygen levels were dropping while I was sleeping, and they wanted to check for fluid in my lungs—another terror to add to the list. Thankfully, one compassionate nurse helped me calm down by explaining what happened. She stayed through her shift and truly made an effort to treat me like a person, not just a patient. That evening, after three days in the hospital, my water broke, and the contractions began. I was exhausted, but we worked all day to get the baby started. During my almost four days at the hospital, I was only three centimeters dilated by Saturday night. The plan was to recheck in the morning, and if I weren't more than four centimeters, we'd do a C-section delivery.

I was up early as we confirmed we'd be moving forward with a cesarean. The next step was an epidural. The head anesthesiologist brought well-worn dad jokes that helped start the morning with a lightness I hadn't felt in days. Throughout my stay, I had explained to the various doctors why I was lying on my side, and this was no different. "I can't lie on my back because it makes me dizzy." Regardless of my explanation, the team insisted I lay on my back. I refused. They attempted to compromise with, "But we only need five minutes." Again, I said no. "One minute?" *No.* Finally, after much cajoling, I agreed to thirty seconds, confirming we'd adjust if I started to feel light-headed. Later, Tom described what he had seen from across the room: within seconds of me laying back, my hands flew up, my skin went white, and my head dropped. A doctor must have hit a crash button because people poured into the room. I came to with at least ten doctors and nurses buzzing around me, and Doctor Dad Jokes growing instantly serious. The thought was that I had experienced a seizure, but it was quickly confirmed that I had just fainted. "I told you so," I muttered under my breath. Thankfully, they followed my suggestion and completed the epidural as I lay on my side.

With this new information and my inability to be laid on my back, the team realized the cesarean surgery had to be done a little differently. The delivering doctor that morning came in to discuss the plan; I was relieved that he was not only understanding of my situation and willing to work with me to make the surgery successful for both of us, but he said he knew me through working with my oncologist. He had been on her team while she deliberated my case—a beautiful connection tying this journey together. He was kind and comforting; his energy instantly put me at ease. I also realized our favorite nurse had swapped shifts to help with the delivery. As they rolled me down the hall into the surgery suite, I knew I was in good hands.

"If you pass out again, we'll put you in a medically induced coma," a nurse said matter-of-factly, and then proceeded with her other tasks. Any comfort I had eased into was ripped away with those few words. I looked to Tom to confirm I had heard her correctly; his helpless, blank stare mirrored my own. I squeezed my eyes shut, willing my body into submission. I grabbed Tom's arms and pulled my face and body toward him, twisting at my ribs just enough to keep me conscious and ready for surgery. I could feel the muscles tearing through my shoulders and back as I clawed to hold on. I knew the ache would haunt me, but the fear of missing my baby being born was unbearable. My jaw was clenched tight, and only whimpered responses were escaping from me as the doctors proceeded.

I could feel them working around me. I could feel the pressure as they opened my skin, and I was grateful for my doctor's recommendation to cut through my past surgery scar not to create further scarring. I willed myself to open my eyes. *This is happening and you need to be here for it. This is happening and you need to stay conscious for it.* In that moment, I scraped the sides of my empty stores for any meager crumbs of energy. I focused on staying awake. I was so focused, I barely registered when they brought a tiny baby to my face. *Open your eyes! See your baby! He's here!* I forced it then, slowly letting in the bright lights. I tried to cry. I tried to feel anything except laser-focused fear. I was there, but the only proof I kissed his tiny little head are the photos our incredible nurse took on her phone for us. *I love you.* I whispered then shut my eyes tight again, afraid it would all fade into black if I didn't turn out the lights myself.

Deep breath in. Slow breath out. I blinked my eyes open as we got ready to roll back to our room. I hesitantly released my white knuckle grip on Tom and flattened my right shoulder. Once the baby was out of me, I could lay on my back without any issues. Hooray. After months of contorting my body, looking directly up at the ceiling felt refreshing.

I was reunited with my little buddy that afternoon, and we immediately fell into a rhythm. Holding him to my heart didn't even feel close enough. My sweet miracle baby boy Parker.

Soon, they moved us to the recovery area, and we spent five more long days in another COVID room at the end of the hall. While we still couldn't accept visitors, the check-ins were constant. Every few hours, a knock at the door to check my vitals, his breathing, my incision, his feeding, my bleeding, his jaundice—it went on and on. The door to the bathroom screeched as it opened. One morning, we woke up to construction and drilling vibrations outside our hospital room window. When we weren't kept awake by the din, we were alone, feeling like someone had forgotten about us in our far-away corner. We still weren't allowed to leave the room, so I could only pace the short distance between the bed and the bathroom, leaving my imprint on the tile floor from all the wear.

And then one morning, after hours of bargaining and pacing, they signed our discharge paperwork. It was April Fools' Day, and I was a viper ready to strike if this was some cruel joke. But, after ten days of quarantine and recirculating air, rules and tubes, and constant monitoring, they just let us . . . walk out. At that moment, driving home, with a tiny hand wrapped around my finger, witnessing his curious eyes watch the rowhouses passing by, I finally felt free to breathe.

We welcomed home life and the wild schedule of a new baby with open arms. While our apartment seemed to be closing in around us as we gained baby gear and gifts, we reveled in the closeness of our little nest. Our family and friends finally met Parker and were awed, just as we were. We took walks, we frequented Target, and we tried to sleep.

I was recovering well from surgery but had some spotting, which I was told was normal. However, cramps and spotting had increased by the end of April, which was not. I reluctantly checked back into the hospital as they tried to help me end the pain and bleeding. Tom held Parker as I pumped from the uncomfortable bed, so he at least had a bottle, while the doctor tried to pull the clots out of me. After confirming it wasn't placenta or pregnancy debris and the bleeding calmed down, they let me go home. I was to call the team if I passed a clot as large as my palm or if I soaked through a pad in an hour. Looking back, of course, I didn't soak through a pad because I kept running to the bathroom. I was tired, but the bouts of lightheaded cabin-pressure feeling were short-lived, and I slept in between feedings. Then I woke up to Tom shaking me on our bathroom floor. "Are you OK?! You passed out!" I blinked once, then twice, and decided to deny it. "No, I didn't. I'm fine," I tried to get up but instantly fainted again. We knew something was wrong but didn't know what to do. Tom had enough brain power to call 911, and that's how, on my first Mother's Day as an actual mother, I rolled out of our apartment on a stretcher headed for the ER instead of brunch.

The emergency room doctors confirmed I had lost an extensive amount of blood. My hemoglobin was at level four (the healthy level is twelve).

A blood transfusion saved my life and brought back the color I hadn't realized I'd lost. By this time, Parker was home with Tom and had to learn to alternate between what little breast milk I could get to him and formula. I was alone again, feeling every bit of the separation when, to my surprise, my delivery doctor walked in, as he was doing his ER rotation. The familiar face and introduction to his kind coworker helped me keep my PTSD at bay as they admitted me to the hospital once again.

My body seemed to be gathering unique ailments like collectible cards. They discovered my cervix was somehow still dilated over a month after Parker's birth and my uterus was full of blood. We tried everything and talked to every doctor. One doctor and I even tried to scrape it out, which was as painful and disgusting as it sounds. I felt the echo of all my former selves, just wanting to be freed, just wanting to fix what was wrong with my body, and move forward with my life. We were all beyond grateful when they discovered I had a loose blood vessel at the top of my uterus that was causing the problem. As we discussed the particulars of the procedure that was going to fix it, I imagined a tiny inflatable tube man wearing a painted smile and flailing arms doing a wacky little dance in there. As quickly as they had discovered the fix, they scheduled me in a surgery suite to complete our plan—I should have had a frequent flier card for that hospital by now. It seemed incredibly appropriate that the foam the medical team used to seal my insides was what military medics use on wounded soldiers to keep them from bleeding out when at war. I limped home, war-weary, happy to have survived another battle.

Throughout the years I've powered through emboldened by action and hope but my fears were always waiting patiently nearby. I created walls to keep them confined but the cage started cracking under the pressure of such relentless prisoners. Restorative practices like therapy, acupuncture, pottery, and meditation have helped a slow release along the way but recently I've been facing the true enormity of what I've been through. After finding and settling into our new home, embracing the simple pleasures of quiet days, regaining some body autonomy after sixteen months of breastfeeding, and celebrating Parker's second birthday, I slowed enough to let my guard down and the cage burst open.

After two more major panic attacks, I started medication to help with my blood pressure and anxiety and I'm happy to say I can feel myself moving forward and mending. I know that nothing is guaranteed, not this moment or the next, but instead of letting that shut me down, I'm allowing it to crack me open. I'm learning it can all live together—the joy, the heartache, the happiness, and the fears.

I believe our lives are made up of a series of moments and some are so big they brand you for life. Even as the scars fade over time and we grow past them, they will always be a part of us with all their pain and beauty. Looking in the mirror, I still sometimes feel anger and sadness when I see my scars, but I also welcome a deep gratitude. I have so much love for this body that carries me. This body that has kitchen dance parties, plays hide and seek among the trees, plants native flowers for the butterflies, and turns mud into mugs. And maybe most importantly, love for the body that holds space not only for my past selves and their scars, but for the person I'm discovering I am today. I've stopped grabbing and rushing toward some future life so I can be here for her and this magnificent moment she and I worked so hard for.

Maybe she's behind the pottery wheel. Maybe she's hiking with the family. But all Kate Rowe really wants to do is share joy with those around her. In the middle of her career in nonprofit marketing, sharing the benefits of play and aquatic exploration, two battles with ovarian cancer shifted her perspective and her body. After life-saving surgeries and with the help of IVF, Kate became the mom of a wonderful, equally joyful child who is schooling her in sharing her "energy" with others, even when they're exhausted. During her fertility journey, Kate rediscovered her love of pottery and has been throwing ever since. As a professional ceramic artist, Kate loves getting her hands dirty and creating inspiring, useful pieces to bring beauty to everyday life. Kate lives in Maryland with her family, and enjoys neighborhood walks among the trees. You can connect with Kate on Instagram @katekatebear.

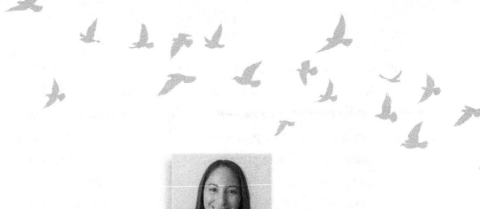

IF NOTHING IS WRONG, THEN HOW DO WE FIX IT?

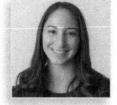

Samantha Bonizzi

I opened my groggy eyes, struggling to focus on the recovery room ceiling. I was flat on my back on a stretcher in my fertility clinic's surgical center. As the bright lights brought me back to the setting, I felt equal parts delirium and anticipation. Just moments ago, I had been ushered into the procedure room and directed to lie down on a table and place my feet in stirrups attached to the end, all so the doctor could suck out as many eggs as possible from my ovaries. Alone, waiting for my nurse to share the outcome, I felt like I was caught inside a weird game of truth or dare. I had dared to lie down, so the eggs could be sucked up into the doctor's vacuum, and then had to wait for them to come back to me, to tell me the truth. I moved my head a few times to shake free the cobwebs caused by anesthesia when the nurse came toward me from behind the curtain. In her hand, she clutched a piece of paper that contained the truth. I held my breath as she handed it to me—it contained my egg retrieval count. The nurses explained that this protocol helped maintain privacy amongst the dozen women I was sharing this room with who were undergoing the same procedure. I opened the folded paper, read the number silently to myself, and exhaled in relief. It was a number that we were hoping for. I whispered a silent thanks to whoever was listening. Things had finally gone according to plan for the first time in this journey.

Adding to the truth, it took me a long time to come to terms with becoming an IVF patient. Before my husband Chris and I set out to have our first child, there wasn't any indication that having a baby would be a struggle for us. We got pregnant so quickly the first time; I believed we were one of the lucky ones.

We found out we were pregnant just a couple of months into trying and were thrilled with the news, especially after getting a false positive just a month prior. The truth was in the blood test I got at my doctor's office— we were *really* pregnant this time. Out of an abundance of caution, and maybe so that we didn't just jinx the whole thing, we waited until around week nine before we began telling our families and close friends. It felt wonderful to share and have them join in our happiness. Our parents were all so excited! Plans were underway as we discussed welcoming the first grandchild on both sides of the family. One of my favorite moments in revealing our special news was when we flew out to San Diego to share, in person, with my grandmother, who we lovingly refer to as Mama, that she would be a great-grandmother. I carefully selected the perfect gift to portray this message and settled on a Little Words Project bracelet that said Great Mama. Other family members gathered around as I gave her the bracelet, and we all witnessed an eighty-year-old woman jump for joy at the revelation.

At thirteen weeks, we naively went in for our prenatal genetic testing. When we saw the baby come up on the screen, we were so excited to lay eyes on our little one that we hardly noticed that the technician had gone quiet. We were laughing and joking as we tried to sneakily take a video of the ultrasound with our phone for my aunt, who had asked us to send her one. The laughing stopped abruptly when the technician announced she had to get the doctor. At that moment, reality began to sink in. As the doctor entered our room, the silence was deafening. "I'm sorry, there is no heartbeat." He confirmed our worst nightmare in those six words.

We had a miscarriage. We had to repeat this truth over and over to our family and friends. They were words I never thought I would have to say, and no matter how many times I had to say them, they kept tearing our whole world apart. I dreaded telling my grandmother after witnessing how happy she was that a baby was on the way. I couldn't face the conversation yet, so I had my mom deliver the unfortunate news. Weeks later, once we had finally caught up on what happened, she asked me if she could still wear her Great Mama bracelet. But I couldn't look at it, so I told her, "Please take it off. Truthfully, I can't stomach seeing it right now. I know there will be a day when I will be able to look at it again, but until then, please do not wear it." She understood, but I think the conversation deepened the loss for both of us.

Five weeks had passed since I had been to the doctor, so I had no idea when the miscarriage occurred, and no one could tell me. The thought that I could have been carrying our dead baby around inside me for weeks haunted me like a sad dream. My mind was filled with so many questions, I thought it might short-circuit. There was no time for answers because we had to figure out what to do with the lifeless being inside me. We opted to have a D&C procedure, which required surgery to remove the tissue from my uterus. The day before the procedure, I had to go to the hospital to get cleared—a daunting task as I was still overcoming the shock of what had happened. While I went through the motions of what I needed to do, my mind was still replaying everything, trying to understand where it all went wrong. As I sat there, numb, the nurse ticked through the required questions, and I went on autopilot. I couldn't believe my first time setting foot in the hospital as a pregnant woman wasn't for the delivery of our baby, but rather because the baby had died before getting the chance to live. Chris came with me for the procedure and my aunt, who worked in the hospital, was also there, making sure I received the best care. As I lay in the hospital bed, Chris on my left and my aunt on my right, I still couldn't process what was happening. Chris adjusted my pillow and then grabbed my hand. My aunt whispered words of encouragement, "You'll get through this . . . it's all going to be OK." When it came time to remove the life that never was, I was surprised at how easy the whole thing went. But even more, I was surprised at how hollow and empty I felt after.

I didn't know until that day that grief has many layers. I understood that I would grieve the loss of my baby—that was easy to grasp. But beyond that, there was this bottomless feeling of pain that took over, once I realized I didn't know the direction my life was heading. Chris and I were at the stage where we were starting to make plans and envision what life would be like. Before the miscarriage, we had stolen away for a few days to celebrate our anniversary in upstate New York. We took the trip midweek in late March, so the area we stayed in was quiet and peaceful and gave us every opportunity to slow down and connect. It was perfect. We spent time hiking and being in nature, which allowed us to dream and talk about our future family. We chatted affectionately about what our child might be like and how we hoped to raise him or her. We left the trip feeling more ready than ever. All that dreaming created a bubble of happiness we floated around inside until that day at the doctor's office. Pop! It was all gone faster than we could have imagined.

The emptiness of our house echoed the emptiness in my heart. Chris and I had been preparing to bring life into our home and suddenly had no idea when that would happen. We had always considered getting a dog but decided to wait and have kids first. That changed in the aftermath of our loss. I could no longer stand the silence that bounced off the walls of what should have been the nursery and lobbied heavily for a puppy to help us endure the loss. We found a breeder nearby with mini bernedoodles described as therapy dogs; that sounded exactly like what we needed. We were the last pick of the litter, and that felt symbolic somehow—like I could trust whichever dog was left was meant to be ours. When we met her one morning in May, she greeted us with puppy kisses, a fast-wagging tail, and an overall sweet and sunny disposition. We decided Sunny was the perfect name for her; we could tell she'd be bringing us the sunshine we needed amidst our rain storm. While Sunny didn't replace what we lost, she brought us immense joy, and caring for her gave us a new purpose.

As we slowly came out of the fog of the miscarriage, Chris reminded me that while we experienced a setback, a family was still within our reach. Chris was vital in getting me through that time, and I felt his love as I had never felt it before. He was patient with me whenever we discussed the loss—always giving me space to share my feelings without judgment— and carved out time to be with me in whatever capacity I needed him, whether it was taking a long walk or simply lying with me when the emotions got too intense. He was gracious with my timeline, showing compassion when I needed to shut out the world, yet was the first one at my side when I was ready to feel like a person again. With his support, I could start to think about trying for a baby again.

The doctors had initially told us that it was not our fault, it was a chromosomal abnormality that had caused the miscarriage, which was further proven when they tested the tissue removed with the D&C.

These things happen. We would hear that over and over again. *It was not a pregnancy you would have wanted, so it self-imploded.* While the doctors meant to be reassuring, I felt more confused about what went wrong. *Miscarriages are more common than you think,* they said, *one in four pregnancies. Keep trying.*

So we did. Keep trying. We took the doctor's advice, and we started trying again as soon as I was physically able. I quickly moved past the physical trauma of watching blood clots pass through me despite having a D&C and the emotional toll of losing a dream that felt so within reach. I set my sights on changing our fate. Sure enough, as the wounds were still healing, we were pregnant. It had only been three months.

No one tells you that the feeling of your first loss will continue, even after they remove that little life and you are expected to move on. Not only is the joy snatched right out from under you, but the taking keeps on taking; you're robbed of a lot of things when you deal with pregnancy after loss. The joy of a positive pregnancy test is no longer available because once you see that positive sign it's impossible to believe anything is true. The excitement of a first ultrasound is shrouded in trepidation because during the last visit in that room, your whole world fell apart. The delight of sharing the news with others gets caught in the lump that takes up residence in the back of your throat; it's made up of fear and anxiety that you'll jinx things if you say "We're pregnant!" too soon. While there's still an underlying happiness, you cannot trust it. Not even a heartbeat can override the fear and anxiety that history may repeat itself.

Even though we had lost our naivety and these nagging, fearful thoughts swirled inside me, I still had hope—and I still believed—it would not happen again. Even as the doctor flagged concerns with things like the fetal heart rate, I kept thinking about the facts: the chances of recurrent miscarriages were so slim. According to the American College of Obstetricians and Gynecologists (ACOG), about 5 percent of women have two or more consecutive miscarriages. I had already paid my dues. There was no way I would be one of those 5 percenters.

After a grueling waiting period at the doctor's office during our eight-week mark (Chris's hand still hasn't recovered from my grip), we found out that it was not a viable pregnancy. I crumbled into Chris's arms and gave in to the heavy sobs as the doctor stood there in silence, waiting. I was, in fact, on the other side of that statistic. I was the 5 percent.

How could this happen to us AGAIN? I somehow navigated my way home alone, repeating this thought in the silence of an empty car, since Chris had to go directly to work. I got home and curled into a ball, unable to think of anything other than how unlucky we were, plain and simple. Or was there something else at play? The first miscarriage had felt random; the second time, though, felt personal. I immediately felt like I was being punished for something or that life was testing me in some way, and the realization set in that I was facing a much bigger hurdle than I could have ever imagined.

I didn't grieve the second loss like I did the first one, or at least not in the same way. While I still felt sadness, it was the overwhelming feeling of anger that engulfed me. I was partly angry with my doctor as I grappled with whether I had rushed into another pregnancy due to his guidance, but I was also undeniably angry with my body; it had failed me once again. It was clear there was something wrong with me since I couldn't hold on to a pregnancy. I was no longer dealing with just a sporadic, random miscarriage. Google searches confirmed what I knew to be true: there must be some underlying issue causing these miscarriages to happen. It was both shameful and enraging.

In the following weeks, as a part of my healing journey, I met with a psychic for a womb and spirit baby reading. I have always believed in the existence of spirit babies and being able to connect to the soul of an unborn child, and prior to meeting with the psychic I had sought connection through meditation and journaling. So when someone who'd experienced loss herself recommended this psychic to me, I knew it'd be a powerful experience aligned with my beliefs. This psychic's practice intends to prepare a woman to become aligned with her inner mother, welcome her spirit baby authentically, remove worries and fears, and heal the inner child by integrating psychic reading, tarot, and other spiritual healing modalities. One of the most telling things the psychic communicated was that she could sense this was the most emotion I've ever experienced in my life. I had to agree with her, as I had never endured a loss or trauma like this before. When she called my spirit, she felt like she was in the middle of the ocean, waves rocking her, water consuming her body. This sentiment was also true; I had never grieved so hard or had this big a challenge to face, and it felt all-consuming—like I was drowning. She also noticed that a different layer of rage sunk in after the second miscarriage and that it had a tight grip on my energy.

The psychic felt strongly that the same spirit baby was trying to come through consistently, which explained why I got pregnant quickly the second time. This realization helped my grief because I didn't feel like I had to say goodbye to my babies. Instead, I could believe it was a delayed reunion, and this spirit baby would continue trying to get to us. I set my sights on fixing whatever was happening with us so we could finally unite with our spirit baby. I used the anger to light a fire inside of me and illuminate our path to each other.

I decided I needed to immediately see a reproductive endocrinologist to receive a full workup for recurrent pregnancy loss—which resulted in me being poked and prodded for months. I threw myself into research, lifestyle changes, testing, and doctor visits. Endless conversations with professionals became a coping mechanism. The pain didn't feel quite so intense when I was taking action. I compiled the best possible team, changing fertility clinics once, doctors twice, and acupuncturists three times to ensure I felt as comfortable as I could feel. While to some, it may have looked like I was taking it overboard at points, my therapist assured me that it was a healthy and expected response to trauma.

I will admit that I had tunnel vision during this time. I was laser focused on making the appropriate changes and getting the best care, and wasn't great about letting Chris in. Because I navigated most of this alone, he grew fearful that I was doing too much and perhaps not fully processing what had happened. As a result, we were in a collision about how to approach our path forward. He urged me to listen to doctors when I insisted on a more research-based approach, which meant advocating for more testing and changing my diet, supplements, and environment. This turbulence was starkly different from what we had gone through after the first loss, when we had come together, leaning on one another. In the aftermath of the first loss, I relied on Chris and his love and support to carry me through that dark time. It had made us stronger. In the aftermath of our second loss, it felt like we were losing each other—I was going one way, and he was going the other.

I wanted him to trust me to take control—it was my body, after all—but I had failed to see that we were still a team. I can't say what eventually brought us back; maybe the realization that we were both working towards the same goal and chose to meet somewhere in the middle? Whatever it was, it worked. Chris got on board with some of the tests I was proposing and my lifestyle changes. I worked harder to prioritize him and our marriage through better communication and efforts to spend time with him and Sunny. We were both willing to do everything in our power to prevent a future miscarriage because we could not fathom going through it again, and we needed each other every step of the way.

After months of comprehensive testing, the doctors concluded our miscarriages were due to bad luck or poor egg quality. While I knew I should have been happy that there wasn't a glaring issue, something about it being purely bad luck was hard to sit with. Without a cause, we didn't have a clear path forward or know how to fix it. IVF was an option since genetic testing could help us decrease the chance of miscarriage, but I struggled with whether it was the right path for us.

The lack of answers also catapulted me into feelings of guilt. If there wasn't a medical cause, I must have done something at one point in my life that deserved this sort of karma. Like *Alice in Wonderland*, I fell down the rabbit hole and spiraled through many levels of "Why me? What did I do to deserve this?" I witnessed friends, family members, old classmates, acquaintances, and coworkers have children, and while I wouldn't wish my situation on anyone, it hardly seemed fair.

As women, we often carry the heavy weight of the conception experience on our shoulders. Maybe it's the lack of what we carry in our bellies that causes us to take this burden on, or it's just that society expects us to. When conception fails, the medical system makes us feel defective. This was fully illustrated when a doctor refused to test Chris's sperm while testing me for everything under the sun. With every blood draw, my guilt and anger towards my body deepened. My bruised ego challenged my womanhood because I could not do the *one* thing that I was supposedly put on this Earth to do. As if that wasn't enough, I added even more guilt to my plate because I was letting those around me down, especially our families. Not only did I fail to deliver a child, but also a grandchild, a great-grandchild, a niece, a nephew.

During another upstate trip Chris and I took, this time with Sunny, I did a lot of self-reflection around my guilt. Sitting around the warmth of the campfire, with Chris cooking our dinner over the open flame and Sunny running around the campsite, I felt happy. But that was quickly chased with feelings of guilt as I ruminated on whether I should feel happiness just yet with all that we were dealing with. I recoiled at another layer of guilt—just add it to the list. This forced me to take the time and reflect. As I sat there in nature with my little family, I could see things more clearly, and I realized that if I was going to make it through this, I had to figure out how to experience, evaluate, and release these layers of guilt. But how? I tried looking outside of myself. The unfortunate truth is that there are so many women struggling—I wasn't alone in this. It dawned on me that perhaps I could unlock my guilt by connecting with these other women and hearing their stories. By relating to their struggles and hearing how they emerged on the other side. Maybe the remedy for guilt was hope. It wasn't easy, but I would find solace in connecting with other women who had experienced fertility challenges as well. Once I realized I was not alone in this, I found I could overcome some of those negative emotions.

But first, I had to make these new connections because I did not have anyone in my immediate circle who had been through anything remotely similar. It was quite the opposite—karma really let me have it when I looked around and realized I had the most fertile group of friends *ever*. As much as they tried to be there for me, their lives were a constant reminder of what I did not have, so there were moments when I had to distance myself to protect my heart. As a lifelong people pleaser, missing the baby showers, removing myself from the group chat where baby pictures were constant, and avoiding events where kids were present made me overly worried about what people would think about my absence. However, I feared that if I did go, they would feel like they needed to walk on eggshells around me and that I might bring down the mood with my grief. Over the holidays, some of my friends had gotten together for brunch with their kids, and I knew one of the girls would be sharing the news of her pregnancy with the group. It pained me not to go and be with them during what was supposed to be a joyous and festive time. Ultimately, I had to think about what was best for me, and I felt that I would be most at ease by sitting this one out. Making this decision helped me see that there's no room for people-pleasing on this journey, and I started to figure out how to set boundaries and prioritize only the things I could handle.

My whole life, I've been used to connecting with other women, from sports teams in high school to a sorority in college, which gave me a lasting group of girlfriends. I've always leaned on this, but it felt isolating when I could no longer relate to the women I'd gone through life with— it was disorienting, and I felt lost. I started paying more attention to the social media accounts focused on pregnancy loss and infertility, and I realized that I could use these platforms to create new communities for myself as many offered support groups and other means of connection. While it was hard to sift through the baby noise all over social media, it was worth it when I landed on something aligned with what I was going through, and I found myself having a growing list of women I could turn to, who understood the journey.

There is a sense of camaraderie among women who struggle to get or stay pregnant. One can't quite understand it unless it's been experienced, so those on similar journeys bond quickly. I felt this when I was in the recovery room after my egg retrieval. Though separated by curtains, there was something powerful about the shared experience with the dozen other women in the room that day, you could feel the hopeful energy in the air. It took everything in me to stay on my stretcher when what I really wanted to do was run through the curtains into each woman's space and shout, "You've got this! I'm rooting for you!" Moments like this made me feel less alone. These connections were especially crucial as I approached the decision about whether to do IVF.

I was in awe of the women I spoke with who had taken this path, and I realized that it was not a sign of weakness—which is how I initially perceived it because it wasn't the "natural" route—but one of strength. And after months of trying to figure out all the answers, there was something very comforting about giving up control. If we did IVF, I'd have to rely on the doctors and my medical team and surrender to the process. I was starting to become so burnt out by it all, and I realized that surrendering was my key to survival. There was a week when I was in a new doctor's office every day, and I recognized how much the running around and constant need to stay on top of things was draining me. If I could submit to one medical team and one path forward, I could perhaps persevere.

Even after I knew IVF was our path, we still deliberated for months. At one point, we received the paperwork to review in preparation for a cycle, and I couldn't get through it without sobbing. There were pages and pages detailing each step, medication instructions, as well as the risks involved, and I suddenly felt the immense weight of making such a vast decision after having to sit with a string of so many other choices. Should I change my diet? Is gluten the culprit? Should I do acupuncture? And will my insurance reimburse me if I do? Should I get a second opinion? Or a third and fourth? Should I change doctors? The list was as long as the nights I laid in bed worrying. I had just spent months going in and out of doctors' offices, and I wasn't sure that I was emotionally ready to take this on.

While I won't downplay the amount of thought and research I put into things, deciding to move forward with IVF came down to my intuition, and something I remembered from the psychic's reading. She could see that I had a tight grip on my expectations for a natural pregnancy, and my spirit guides had communicated that opening myself up to a different path could remove the pressure of needing motherhood to happen a certain way. Maybe *how* it happened didn't matter quite so much. I knew I was made for motherhood in my soul, and if I could lead with that belief, maybe everything else would fall into place.

My therapist also helped me see that I had used my gut instincts to guide me during other critical points during this journey and that all of those things had turned out okay. As I considered her observation and what my guides communicated, I realized I had developed a connection to myself and my intuition. There was a power in knowing I could trust myself, what I wanted, and what I knew to be true for me and my path forward to motherhood.

So, I took the plunge.

I did not expect the IVF journey to be incredibly empowering. In one way, I was giving up control, but in another, I understood that I had the power to shape my outcome. Frequent monitoring leading up to the egg retrieval required me to go into the office for blood work and ultrasounds to ensure the medications were working correctly. With this level of involvement, I always felt like I was making progress and working toward something. It gave me purpose. With each blood draw and close-up of my ovaries, I could feel myself getting nearer and nearer to having a baby. These were tangible things based on science. I was no longer questioning and deliberating about what to do next—we were finally in execution mode.

IVF brought Chris and me close together again, another surprise I wasn't expecting. Chris had to administer shots for me every day, which brought about a whole new level of intimacy, and mentally, he became my support system. Before the egg retrieval, the shots had to be administered in my lower abdomen every night at the same time for ten days. As someone who likes to be in control, it was hard to entrust Chris with this critical task. Initially, I'd pepper him with questions like, "Are you sure you have the right amount of liquid in the vial? Is that the right spot, or should it be higher up? Should we watch the video again?" My trust grew as the days progressed, and the experience became second nature; he was a thorough caregiver, and I was the patient.

As we prepped for a transfer, the shots moved to my butt every single morning—and these progesterone-in-oil shots were *no joke*. They hurt like hell, and while I was the one who physically felt the pain every day, Chris would encourage me through it. He'd remind me to ice beforehand or massage the area afterward to help alleviate the sting and would meet me with a big hug on the days when there was more blood than normal.

While I was grateful for the support, any inkling of pain threw me into spirals of disbelief that we had to do this. There was so much we had to endure to have a baby, whereas other people sneeze and get (and stay) pregnant. On the bad days, like when I'd find out someone else in my life was pregnant, I'd feel the "why me?" thoughts start to creep back in.

The results-driven part of IVF can be a mind fuck. There's the constant pressure of advancing to the next level, which gets emotionally taxing. Out of the amount of eggs retrieved, only a certain number mature and fertilize with your partner's sperm. Only a portion of those make it to the embryo stage and through genetic testing, which is why women will go through multiple rounds until they have a number they're comfortable with. Once this is complete, you can finally consider the second phase, the embryo transfer. While this phase is less intensive, it can feel like a lot is riding on it because it does not guarantee a pregnancy.

The waiting through all of this was excruciating; the waiting for the retrieval results (and all of the subsequent phases), the waiting for the transfer, the waiting to find out if I was pregnant, the waiting between appointments, the waiting, the waiting, the waiting. It went on and on, and this was after all of the waiting we had to face through two miscarriages, which kept delaying our future.

I often described this period as being stuck in purgatory. Though Chris and I were ready for the next phase of our lives, we met factors beyond our control that held us back. We had crossed the line into whatever this waiting world was, and there would never be any going back. Meanwhile, it felt like we were forced to watch everyone else pass us by, celebrating as their dreams came true. It just didn't make sense. We never faltered in achieving the next level in any other area of our lives. We got the jobs right out of college, we found the apartment where we wanted to begin our life together, and the wedding, while postponed thanks to COVID-19, finally happened, and it was everything we dreamed. No matter how hard we tried, we couldn't get to the next phase of our lives and start this next chapter.

In a way, I believe I had been waiting to have my own family long before I met Chris. As a child of divorce, I often felt torn between two different worlds. I was the only child of my parents, which often felt lonely. They both remarried and had more children, but they were all much younger than me and hard to relate to. I dreamed of having my own family one day with children who were close in age because I wanted to create the experience I didn't have. With each miscarriage, this dream became further from reality, but one thing remained true: I could protect myself just as I did when I was a little girl.

Looking back, I believe that what I went through as a kid helped me grow and become more self-reliant. I was the only one in the world who understood what I was going through, and therefore, I learned how to persevere and look out for myself. This mindset can have its pitfalls, like not fully letting Chris in because my default is to think I can deal with things by myself, but overall it's made me a stronger person.

I noticed a parallel to what I was experiencing now as an adult. I had to navigate a world that I didn't choose to be in, this time infertility. While I could let myself crumble, I knew there was another path I could choose—the one of growth. The challenges I faced as a kid gave me a powerful sense of self. And the challenges I was facing now could help me fine-tune that sense of self as a woman on her path to motherhood.

The reality of this sunk in once I noticed that things were transcending beyond the fertility world. Something I learned in the doctor's office—advocating for myself—started to take shape in daily life. Previously, if I had been hurt by someone I would have easily let it slide or taken on the responsibility. But I started to stand up for myself and make my feelings known using a newfound confidence.

I realized that it is the journey, not the destination, that matters because it's what builds resilience. I chose to use this waiting period as an opportunity to evolve rather than let it paralyze me. There have been so many choices that I've had to make during this experience. Why not choose to evolve?

A few months after my first miscarriage, I wrote the following in my journal in a letter to my past self, who had just found out about the loss: *You'll have an extremely hard few months ahead. But you'll come out the other side and learn a lot from the experience. You'll be even more wise and emotionally in tune than you are now. You have an incredible support system and a growing number of people (and now a furry friend) to love. You will feel heartbroken for a while, but I promise you will get the will to try again.* These words have never rung truer, and I revisit them during moments of uncertainty.

I'd like to believe that I've gotten through the lowest of lows, but the truth is, I don't know what the rest of this experience will bring. There isn't a baby in my arms and a neat little bow wrapped around my story yet. We're lucky that IVF has been good to us and that we experienced success with both our retrieval and transfer, but I'm still waiting for my happy ending. Even with success, the anxiety follows me like a shadow because I now know how easily things can go awry. While we have a plan, a big part of this is simply out of our hands. The waiting periods still loom, the ultrasounds are still just as scary, sharing a pregnancy with loved ones still feels impossible, and I will have to relive my past traumas at critical moments in my life.

As frightening as all of this is, I know the only way for me to go is THROUGH. I want a baby, so I have to get pregnant again, get through my first trimester, and so on. I must learn how to hold onto the joy and hope alongside the fear and anxiety. There's no sense in trying to push away the negative thoughts. They exist and beg to be acknowledged, and I've learned that is really the only way to take back my power. The best I can do is identify them as they are—for what they are—thoughts. They aren't necessarily my beliefs. Therefore, I will not let them define any present or future pregnancy experience. Again, it comes down to a choice.

I've always been someone who believes that everything happens for a reason. I still do to some degree, but I've given up on finding the reasons. Things happen. It's how we choose to react to them that matters. I'm *choosing* to become stronger from this experience because I know it will make me a better mom when that day finally comes. I've learned how to advocate for myself, set boundaries to protect myself and my future family, and trust my intuition—all things that will help me in motherhood. I also have a calling to serve and support others on a similar journey, which is a new and unexpected path for my life, but one that I am embracing wholeheartedly.

For now, we continue to wait. We wait for this chapter to close, for our spirit baby to finally grace us. We wait, and we wait, and we wait some more. The waiting periods are laced with both fear and hope and depending on the day, one tends to outweigh the other. But I feel in my bones that with each day, I'm getting closer to motherhood. And when that day comes, it will be that much sweeter.

Samantha is a writer with a background in public relations and communications. She spent her early career working in PR for lifestyle brands and has since transitioned to a corporate internal communications role at a tech company. She grew up in New Jersey, where she's lived most of her life (besides a brief stint in New York City), and now resides just outside Montclair with her husband and mini bernedoodle. She loves the area and has written several stories about things to do and places to go for a local lifestyle website, The Montclair Girl. She also loves reading, working out and doing yoga, hiking and being outdoors, as well as traveling. Samantha has always had a passion for wellness and women's health, which has taken center stage in her life since experiencing pregnancy loss and fertility challenges. Now, she wants to pay what she's learned forward and is on a mission to help women who find themselves on similar paths. You can learn more about Samantha and connect with her on Instagram @ sam.bonizzi.

CHASING RAINBOWS

Sarah Goldsborough

Half-naked, I lay shivering on the ice-cold operating table. A question I hadn't thought to ask earlier, suddenly pops into my head as my heart rate slows, and I grow sleepy.

"What will happen to the remains?"

There is a moment of silence and then, "It will be discarded with medical waste." The nurse's cold, clinical reply sent chills up my spine.

A panic rushes over me, but it's too late. The room is closing in on me and the lights grow dim as the anesthesia does its job. This is the last thing I remember, right before drifting off into the darkness as my sixteen-week-old baby is aborted.

This baby was supposed to be our surprise—our happy ending after three miscarriages. She was a plot twist, after deciding we were done trying, right before my fortieth birthday. She had been the sibling our six-year-old son Camden had patiently been waiting for. This was "our girl" and we knew she would complete our family. Looking back, I always knew I'd have a girl. Even before I found out I was pregnant, I would have vivid dreams about her—I knew what she looked like. I consulted with several psychics, who told me all about her during our readings. One in particular, a good friend and client of mine, shared with me during a session that even though we had decided to stop trying, she still saw a girl energy all around me. I remember her saying she was there if we chose to accept her. Otherwise, if we didn't, her soul would move on to another family.

Chose? What the hell does that even mean? If I got pregnant again, why would I not "choose" her? I mulled over this as I left the session. One year later it became painfully clear what it meant.

I found out I was pregnant for the first time in 2013, when my husband Larry and I had only been dating for about four months. Luckily, we had already moved in together and had the marriage talk. The excitement we felt outweighed the shock of finding out we were pregnant so soon. Larry and I strolled into the doctor's office at eight weeks, basking in our naivety. I never imagined that they would deliver anything other than good news that day. Let alone a sucker punch to the stomach: "I don't see a heartbeat, Sarah." All of the air left my lungs when the ultrasound tech ever-so-softly gutted me with those words.

I don't remember much of what the doctor told me that day. I stared at her moving lips, but I couldn't comprehend the words coming out of her mouth. Only thirty minutes before, Larry and I were joking about how the baby was probably going to have a big head, and now the doctor was giving me options for how to proceed with the miscarriage. Talk about a mind fuck.

While our joy was sucked out of our hearts in that moment, I still held on to a feeling that everything was going to be okay. This was our first pregnancy, these things happen, we can try again. Life had always been pretty good to me, I mean, I had been through some shit, but I was strong and it always worked out. I believed in my heart that we would eventually have the positive outcome we were hoping for.

I ended up needing to have a D&C, as many women who have early miscarriages do, to remove all pregnancy tissue safely and to avoid excessive bleeding or infection. During this procedure, the doctor discovered that I had a bicornuate, or heart-shaped, uterus, and there was a wall of cartilage separating it into two compartments. My doctor explained to me that although this was a rare anomaly, it could mean I'd have a more challenging time getting and staying pregnant, but it didn't mean it was impossible. I was advised to keep trying, as getting pregnant didn't seem to be an issue. At the time of this diagnosis, I was wrapped up in my loss. My concern for this discovery was minimal, as my doctors seemed optimistic that it wouldn't be much of a hindrance. In hindsight, I believe this was a major contributing factor to my miscarriages. If I knew then, all the struggles that lie ahead, I would've sought other fertility options from the beginning. A part of me will always be haunted by the roads I didn't take.

About a year later, I found out I was pregnant again.

This pregnancy ended in another early miscarriage. Another D&C. I wasn't sure what this writing on the wall meant, but I began to believe this would be my pattern. My doctors told me to be considered abnormal, I had to have three consecutive miscarriages. I couldn't fathom the feeling of losing yet another one. The weeks following each D&C were some of my darkest days. Excitement was abruptly replaced with emptiness. The life I imagined with my child disappeared. I felt like the dark fog that surrounded me would surely hold me captive forever. I would drive to work in silence, and not remember how I got there, my mind was on autopilot.

Although I had my family and Larry to lean on, they just didn't understand how I was feeling. As life around me continued on, my loneliness grew. In those darkest hours of solitude, I found myself praying; not something I was accustomed to doing very often. My parents had always told me to turn to God in times of need, and although I had never really made that spiritual connection before, I felt like I had no one else to turn to. *God, if you're listening, please help me get through this.* And I believe He did. As time went on, albeit slowly, the fog would dissipate, and the future would start to look bright again.

We got engaged in early 2015 and decided to have a small wedding in September. I found out two weeks before our wedding that I was pregnant again. *Fuck.* Of course, this would happen right before my wedding. As I stared down at the positive pregnancy test I impulsively took in the tiny Walgreens restroom, all I could see was me being robbed of yet another joy: my wedding day. I couldn't imagine why my third pregnancy wouldn't go the way the other two had. These losses were infiltrating every part of my life.

A few days before our wedding, I started bleeding, which was new. The past miscarriages had never been symptomatic. But, it solidified what I already knew was happening; I was losing another pregnancy.

"There's nothing I can do now," I sighed to my fiancé as I continued finalizing wedding arrangements. "I just hope the worst is over before the wedding." We were headed out of town for our nuptials, and then on to Hawaii for our honeymoon.

I don't have time for this. I made a doctor's appointment for the week we returned from Hawaii.

Over the next week, the bleeding went away as quickly as it came, and I felt fine for the most part—not much cramping or any symptoms of a miscarriage. I was just super tired; but planning a destination wedding and all the festivities that accompany it is exhausting. I figured I had experienced an early miscarriage, and luckily, the bleeding had gone away before our big day. Thank God.

Our first day in Hawaii, we hiked to the top of Diamond Head, an inactive volcano. Afterward, I decided to lie down for a much-needed nap before dinner. I didn't wake up until the following day. I told my husband that the six-hour time change had thrown me off. "I can finally relax, after all the stress and excitement from the past few weeks," I said as I perused the room service menu for breakfast.

We had an amazing honeymoon, despite me getting seasick on a snorkeling excursion, and my sudden aversion to the Mai Tai's I had been looking forward to drinking. One evening, as we watched a spectacular Hawaiian sunset over dinner and drinks, something suddenly dawned on me. As I sat there nursing my watered-down cocktail, the tranquil ukulele music filling the air, the thought that I might still be pregnant popped into my head. I looked at my husband across the table, enjoying his third or fourth drink, and I just smiled. With the amount of bleeding I had before the wedding, there was a good chance it would probably still end up being a miscarriage. We would know in a few days when we returned home, so no sense bringing it up at this beautiful moment, spoiling the mood.

The morning we were scheduled to return home, I woke up feeling anxious. All of the wedding and honeymoon festivities were ending, and it was time to return to reality. An indescribable sense of dread came over me. I wasn't ready to face another miscarriage, and throughout our honeymoon, I hadn't been able to keep my mind off the fact that I might have to have another D&C. The fact that this would be our third one meant we would most likely have to start thinking about other options to have a baby. I just wanted to pull the 1000-thread-count covers up over my head and sink into that Hawaiian hotel bed forever.

Later that morning, as we were getting ready to leave the hotel, we looked out an expansive window by the elevator on the twentieth floor that overlooked Waikiki Beach. The view took my breath away. Right over the ocean was the most magnificent rainbow stretching as far as the eye could see. Although rainbows are common in Hawaii, this was the first one we had seen all week. Looking back, I believe it was a sign for what was to come.

I begrudgingly filled out the paperwork in the waiting room of my OB-GYN's office, checking off the box that declined our right to receive genetic testing blood work. I was thirty-four, just shy of being considered a geriatric pregnancy. *God, I can't stand that term.* Each year after thirty-five, the chances of genetic abnormalities increase significantly, so testing is highly recommended. But honestly, those things were the least of my worries. I was okay with whatever God wanted to give me. As I finalized the paperwork with my signature and date, I realized it probably didn't matter anyway, because it would be business as usual. They were going to tell me there was no heartbeat, and everything I had already been prepared for would be confirmed.

As I lay on the same godforsaken table that had become a sort of graveyard, I focused on the ceiling and rehearsed my reaction to the news that would be coming. I couldn't look at the monitor and witness another lifeless, peanut-shaped fetus for a third time. I had gotten to know the ultrasound tech; I work with people, and have a knack for connection. Even in the midst of all the sadness, I was able to break through her stoic way, and feel her care. *It must suck to be the bearer of bad news.* As I lay there on my back, searching the ceiling for a focal point, I wondered how she was able to get up and deliver these blows to women day after day.

"Don't beat around the bush; just tell me if it's bad news," I told her flatly. I was ready to get the whole thing over with.

She started the exam, and I held my breath as I stared at the same little speck on the tiled ceiling. It felt like it was taking an eternity. I couldn't help myself and glanced over at her face; her expression was different from the last two times we had met in this tiny room of doom. The light from the screen illuminated her surprise, and I thought I could see confusion in her eyes as she moved the Doppler device around, listening for a heartbeat.

"Oh my God, what? Just tell me!" I didn't know what this confused look meant; I just knew it was different.

Right as I was about to diagnose my third miscarriage, the unfamiliar sound of excitement filled the room. It was the most beautiful sound I've ever heard in my life. "That's your baby's heartbeat. You're pregnant!" She had a massive smile on her face as she turned the screen toward me so I could see.

I stared at the bright screen and must have looked like a deer caught in headlights, as I watched and listened to my ten-week-old baby's heart flutter like a little butterfly. We both laughed with happy tears in our eyes.

Holy shit. I was sure she was going to tell me I was having another miscarriage, so I had not prepared for this. The emotions I felt in that moment can only be described as divine. I have never been a super religious person, but the moment I saw my baby's heartbeat, I intuitively knew God was with me. And I knew I was in the midst of a miracle. They never could explain why I had been bleeding, but instead assured me everything looked just fine. In that moment, I felt a calm wash over me that I had never experienced before. I knew in my soul that my baby and I were protected.

On May 7, 2016, my son Camden arrived exactly one week late; very on brand for the stubborn, sleepy little Taurus I've come to know and love. He was a ray of sunshine from the moment he was born. He was only a few days old when he smiled at my husband and I for the first time, and he hasn't stopped smiling since. Camden is truly a beautiful, happy child. He's a rainbow in human form. It's hard to remember what life was like before he was with us. Having him changed me in so many ways. Becoming a mother gave me a newfound sense of purpose. Everything I did after he was born was to make sure he had the happiest life I could give him. The love I felt for him massively outweighed the pain of my prior miscarriages; they made me all that more grateful for him.

That's the thing about life—it can be truly unpredictable. I came to know this well, with each of my pregnancies. I realized pretty quickly, I had very little control—of anything. I had spent my life preparing for the calm waters, only to have the unforeseeable tempest of miscarriage come along and knock me off course. And just as I became accustomed to weathering the storm, God gave me a rainbow. I discovered I had a choice: I can fight what is out of my control, or I can surrender to it. For me, finding acceptance in the fact that I had very little control over the outcome of my pregnancies was key, not only for finding more joy during my pregnancies, but for healing after each loss.

After each miscarriage, I allowed myself to feel all of the emotions. I allowed the darkness to roll in like a thick fog, because it was going to find a way in regardless. Eventually, the fog would lift, and I was able to move forward. Letting go of control, or some may say, having faith in God's plan, allowed me to be more present with each of my pregnancies, regardless of their potential outcome. With Camden, my only full-term pregnancy, I was so grateful for every little kick I felt in my belly, and for countless tiny moments after he was born. I understand now why birth is called a miracle. In my case, it definitely was.

Although my pregnancy with Camden was fairly easy and uneventful, I had some complications during his birth and immediately after. When he was only eight weeks old, I had to have an emergency abdominal surgery to remove an ovarian cyst and subsequently, one of my ovaries. My doctor was aware of the cyst before I became pregnant with Camden, but believed it to be small and noncancerous. We agreed they would monitor it every six months. Unbeknownst to me and my doctor, it had grown to the size of a football by the time I gave birth to my son. It ended up rupturing two months after I gave birth and landed me in the hospital for five days, without Camden.

So much could've gone wrong while I was carrying Camden, as the cyst weighed more than him when he was born. Had it ruptured while I was pregnant, there's a good chance both of us would've died. It was truly a miracle that nothing happened until after he was born. Without a shadow of a doubt, I believe it was by the grace of God and his protection that prevented the cyst from rupturing, giving us both our beautiful lives.

After my emergency abdominal surgery, despite the excruciating physical pain, I did find some comfort laying in my hospital bed, believing the worst was over. No one had ever talked to me about the extreme anxiety that would wake me up in the middle of the night, strangling me from my sleep, flooding my mind with fearful intrusive thoughts that I didn't know were lurking inside me. I couldn't sleep, I couldn't eat—I was overcome with this terror that something was going to happen to Camden because I was not there to protect him. "My baby needs me!" I sobbed into the phone to my mother as I tried in vain to pump breast milk in between bouts of debilitating post-operative pain.

Not being able to hold Cam or breastfeed him when I got home from the hospital devastated me. I had fought like hell to survive, but still, that didn't feel like enough. I couldn't give him what I felt he needed most, and that meant I was a failure as a mom. The anxiety worsened to the point that I was having daily panic attacks. I was terrified something bad was going to happen to Camden, or to me. I was convinced one of us was going to be abducted at the mall or at Target, as I had heard horror stories of that happening. My love of watching true crime, paired with postpartum anxiety, proved to be a toxic mix for me. With the exception of going to work, I barely left the house. I would have vivid daydreams of people holding Camden and dropping him down the stairs, so I became only comfortable with my husband or mom holding him. This exhausting nightmare went on for months.

The postpartum anxiety overpowered my faith that God was watching out for us. Eventually, the constant, uncontrollable worry, spiraling into panic became too much to handle. All of this came to a head one day when I was driving with my mom and Cam to the grocery store, explaining to her how I was having these terrifying visions. Just talking about it immediately sent me right over the edge into one of my panic attacks, and she made me call my doctor right then and there. I went on Zoloft, an antidepressant, to help control the postpartum anxiety. Within a few weeks, I could start to breathe a little easier, and my daily anxiety visits came less often. It didn't take away the anxiety completely, but it helped me manage the debilitating fear and intrusive thoughts that had been wreaking havoc on my life.

When Camden was about eight months old, I found out I was pregnant again. An unfamiliar reaction of fear unfolded in my belly. I'd experienced the fear of impending loss with my previous pregnancies, but as I stared at the positive pregnancy test, I knew this was different. The trauma of my post-birth, near death experience, made me fear getting pregnant again. I hadn't fully processed my feelings about it because I wasn't planning on getting pregnant this soon. I didn't like that I was scared, but my body was still recovering from birth, a major surgery, and I was just starting to get my life back from the anxiety that had been in the driver's seat for far too long.

"It's too soon," I said to my husband when I shared the news with him. I didn't think I could handle it.

I found out at my initial appointment that I had, once again, miscarried. The guilt took over the sadness I should have been feeling. I hadn't been happy about this pregnancy and so I figured God was punishing me for feeling that way. And because of my misplaced happiness, there was a part of me that believed I deserved for this to be one of the worst miscarriages I had experienced yet. The doctor prescribed medication to expel the remains at home, avoiding a D&C. I figured it would be a much better experience, but I was horribly wrong. It was painful and traumatic.

Waking up abruptly in the middle of the night to intense cramping, I barely made it to the toilet to release the fetus. Larry leaves for work at 3:00 a.m., so I was home alone, Cam asleep in his crib. Doubled over from the abdominal pain, I stared between my legs into the toilet, not knowing what to do next. I wiped the tears from my eyes so I could see more clearly. *Was that a fetus floating in the toilet?* My doctor hadn't given me any kind of instructions or warnings. So I sat there, alone, on the toilet, sobbing. Quietly begging, *Please help me, God. I don't know what to do. I'm sorry I wasn't ready for this baby*, I prayed.

After a few minutes, I closed my eyes while tears ran down my face and neck and did what needed to be done. I flushed the toilet.

I'm so sorry. I'm so sorry. I'm so sorry. I wept my apologies up to God, I sobbed as I held my hands over my stomach where the fetus had been and shuttered at the reality that I had just flushed it down the toilet. I moaned my sorries to the babies I had lost, connecting with their little spirits in this dark moment of my own humanity. And lastly, I apologized to myself.

I should've gone on birth control after my surgery. I made my way back to my bed and checked the monitor to see Camden was still sleeping soundly in his bed. My body was obviously not strong enough to carry another baby yet. And I had lost another one.

Looking back, I can honestly say the guilt mothers carry for their miscarriages is the most fucked up part about the whole ordeal. Even though I didn't choose these losses, I somehow believed it was my fault— and only mine—that they had happened. Every morning when I got up, that guilt was the first thing I put on, and I wore it like a weighted vest for a long time. It took years, and a lot of therapy, for me to admit to Larry the loneliness and guilt I felt following each miscarriage. He assumed I had moved on because I stopped talking about it every day. He didn't know that I'd cry in the shower, or in the car, daily for months. No one really knew the extent of my grief, except for God.

During the pandemic, I was forced off work for ten weeks. Larry was an essential worker, so Cam and I were at home most days. Although it felt like *Groundhog Day*, we had fun. I was aware that I'd probably never get to spend that much time with him around the clock ever again, and so I soaked it up.

When Cam turned four that May, Larry and I started discussing having another baby. Cam loved being around other kids, and we knew he'd be an amazing big brother. It had been a few years since my last pregnancy, and a part of me was content with our lives, just us three. But there was another part of me that still wanted to give it another try. One more try for Camden. I've already been through hell and back, so I thought I had nothing to lose. I put the vest of guilt back on and carried around the responsibility of ensuring Camden wouldn't be an only child.

As I contemplated the road ahead, I wondered if this guilt was what propelled people to bring more children into the world, despite how they honestly felt. Did they love having kids so much, or did they just feel an obligation to other people? I wasn't sure what I wanted. Cam was now four, and fairly independent. Did I really want to start all over with the baby phase?

By September 2020, I was pregnant for the sixth time. I actually don't remember much about this pregnancy. Except that, the week I found out I had miscarried, my brother and his wife announced to us that they were expecting baby number two. They weren't aware of my pregnancy or miscarriage, so it was very off-putting when I burst into sobs at their announcement. I had never done that before. Throughout the entirety of my journey through pregnancy and loss, I'd never lost it like that in front of people. It was unexpected. But it was honest. It wasn't censored or polite, because I just didn't have it in me to be that way anymore. I was happy for them, but the overwhelming wondering of "why can't this happen for me?" was the dominating emotion. Sometimes the feelings of sadness would be so overwhelming, the only way to survive them was to self-isolate. More than once, I would be on the tail end of a miscarriage only to find out a close friend was pregnant. I didn't want to dampen their excitement so I would just distance myself.

After my fifth miscarriage, Larry and I decided we were done trying to have another baby. I couldn't subject myself or my family to this emotional roller coaster anymore. In hindsight, I would've been more proactive earlier in my pregnancy journey if I had known how many miscarriages I'd endure—I would've sought help or alternative opinions to those of my OB-GYN's. But at this point, I didn't have it in me to seek other options. The miscarriages had pushed me to my limit. I don't know if it was the realization that I wouldn't have any more children, but I started to wonder if that was something I even wanted.

Before I had Cam, I got lost in a void after each miscarriage, but I would pull myself out, because I knew in my heart, we needed to keep trying. After I had Cam, my life felt so complete. Yes, I would've loved and accepted more children had we been blessed with them, but when I really sat with it, I realized I didn't feel that same void as I did before Cam. And when one sits with the hard realizations, inevitably, the truth begins to surface. I started to wonder if maybe I had been trying to fill a void that wasn't there at all. Part of me could see I had gotten so caught up in the hamster wheel of pregnancy and miscarriage, that I hadn't stopped to ask myself if having another child was chasing after what my heart truly wanted anymore. Had I surrendered so much control amid all of my losses, that I lost sight of the fact that maybe that void had already been filled? As I considered this reframe, I felt content drawing a line in the sand. We were done.

If you want to make God laugh, they say, tell him your plans.

About a year later, one month shy of my fortieth birthday, I found out I was pregnant, yet again. I felt strangely calm going into this pregnancy. I'd accepted that whatever was meant to be, would be. I'd also adopted a detached, carefree attitude, I think as a defense mechanism, due to the disappointment and trauma of repeated miscarriages. I'd tricked myself into thinking I'd be fine no matter the outcome. So, back on the hamster wheel I went.

The vibes were good the day my eight-week ultrasound came along. The ultrasound tech was elated to deliver good news for a change. She was genuinely happy and excited for me. My regular OB-GYN wasn't in the office that day, so she promised to text her the good news. I sat in the room by myself for a moment and stared at the ultrasound photo she had printed out for me. "Hi. We've been waiting for you. Better late than never." In that moment, as the sun beams spilled in through the mini blinds, I made a decision: *No matter what happens, I want to remember the joy I feel in this exact moment.* I sat quietly in the happiness of those thoughts for a few minutes while waiting to talk to the doctor. What we remember in some of our life's most defining moments is funny. I'll always cherish the moments I had that morning; it was as if the sadness that had paved our way to this point had disappeared back into the woods. I wasn't worried about what might come after. I was truly joyful being there in that moment, me and my baby.

This was my first pregnancy since Camden that I had made it past eight weeks, and I decided that I wanted to have the twelve-week genetic testing done since I was now forty. We wanted to make sure everything was okay, before telling Camden that he was going to be a big brother.

I had envisioned the look on his face when we finally told him. I knew it was going to be an extraordinary moment for us all.

Waiting on the genetic testing results felt like the week before Christmas when I was a kid; every day felt like an eternity. I was busy at work and at home, but it was all I could think about. I kept my phone close by, awaiting the call from my doctor's office. Finally, as I was in the middle of highlighting my client's hair, my phone rang. It was the call I'd been waiting for. My heartbeat picked up pace. I knew no matter what they told me, it would be life-changing.

This was it. I would know what my family's future was going to look like in the next few seconds. When I answered, it was the ultrasound tech's familiar voice on the other end. Her tone told me all I needed to know.

It wasn't good.

The genetic testing determined that there was a 98 percent chance that the baby would have Down Syndrome. And just like that, my dream evaporated into a nightmare I couldn't wake up from.

Are you fucking serious?! I wanted to scream into the phone, but all I felt was despair. *How is this happening? Were the five miscarriages not enough?* I could barely swallow the nausea. I had been a fool to think I'd actually have a healthy baby now at forty, after all my years of struggle. In that moment of darkness, I despised the God that had protected Camden and me.

I hadn't planned on asking her the baby's gender that day, but I needed to confirm what I already knew in my heart to be true. "Is it a boy or a girl?" I held my breath as I waited for her to answer.

She paused, then responded, "It's a girl. I'm so sorry, Sarah."

I was having an out-of-body experience. I couldn't see straight; I felt like I was moving in slow motion as I walked out of that break room to finish up with my client. I had entered that tiny room to take the call, as a living person, and walked out a ghost of myself. I was no longer the person I had been before. The remnants of my soul that were left after my previous miscarriages had now been completely sucked out of me, like all the D&Cs I had experienced. I was completely empty inside. I returned to my studio, pushed the soul-crushing news I had just received, down as deep as I could make it go, and acted like nothing had happened as I kept on foiling my client's hair.

A day later, I listened quietly as the genetic counselor went over all the facts, scenarios, percentages, possibilities, and realities of Down Syndrome. In the next week, we were going to have to decide on whether or not we were going to continue on with the pregnancy. Amid this, I remembered what my psychic friend had told me. This was the "choice" she had spoken of. What she failed to mention, was that it was going to be the most challenging goddamn choice I'd ever had to make in my life.

Larry and I walked in conversational circles for days, trying to find a decision we could live with. It was a fork in the road, and no matter our choice, both roads led us to places we did not want to go.

We knew that having a child with Down Syndrome would drastically change the life we had worked so hard to build, and loved so much. We thought about what our lives might look like in the long term. We would most likely care for this child for the rest of their lives. Was that something that we were prepared for? We were given the statistics on how many babies with Down Syndrome need open heart surgery upon birth, as well as how many die early in life, depending on the severity of the myriad of health conditions that are associated with Down's. We were told that we would never be out of the woods with Down

Syndrome. Our child could be fairly healthy one day and present a new health problem the next. What if we had a child that had major health problems or died after a few months or years? What would that do to Cam? How could we give him a sibling only to have it potentially taken away at a young age? Or, on the flipside, perhaps giving him a sibling that would require most of our attention, and what would that do to Cam? A part of me knew that Cam would adapt and be an amazing big brother no matter what we decided. But the amount of anxiety it was already causing me was telling me that this was too much for me to handle. I knew how much stress I had been under when Cam was a baby, and he didn't have any health problems. I knew that if I had this baby, understanding all of the possible health complications, I'd be setting myself up for a long, difficult road. And I was tired of traversing the jagged cliffs of loss and pain. I had picked myself up, over and over again, and figured out how to carry the weight of the losses that never quite goes away. How could I be asked to lose, yet again, and in such a very big way?

Some may say that if you believe in God, he doesn't give you more than you can handle. Or that bad things can happen even to healthy children, so all you can do is trust in God. But I just couldn't get past the fact that the likelihood of significant health problems, or possibly death, was going to be much greater with a child with Down's, with our girl. I didn't want to live my life in a constant state of fear and anxiety. I knew how that would affect my marriage, my health, and the type of mother I'd be. I thought of mothers I knew who were navigating life with a special needs child, and while I admired them very much, I just didn't think I could be that person. And when I got really honest with myself in those hallowed hours alone in the middle of the night, where it was just me and God, I admitted that I didn't want to be that mom.

Ultimately, we decided not to continue with the pregnancy. Once the decision was made, arranging the procedure was the next step. Although the doctors and counselors I spoke to were kind, the whole experience felt shameful. I had the choice to either go to one specific hospital downtown that performed abortions, or I could go to an abortion clinic. They told me I couldn't go to my usual hospital for the procedure because it was Catholic, and they couldn't help me there. The sick heat of shame overwhelmed me and threatened to swallow me whole when I was advised to choose the hospital over the clinic to avoid the pro-life protesters. *The hospital would be much more discreet*; so discreet, in fact, I had to be given special directions, along with a map of the hospital, to find the unmarked door I needed to enter. And due to COVID-19 restrictions, I had to do it alone, once again.

The aftermath of having the abortion was one of the most painful times in my life. People often didn't know what to say or do to show their support. I never had anyone downright condemn me, but the judgment was apparent. People may think they know what they would do in my shoes, but they don't. When I reflect back over this time, I feel how much strength and courage it took to make the choice we made. It was honest. It wasn't people-pleasing. It was what we were able to do in one of the worst moments of our lives—and it was true.

But truth is not a shortcut for the grieving process that went on for a few years. I had to accept our choice, because I knew it was the best thing I could do for our family. But at times, the grief, in all its multifaceted layers, threatened to take me down forever. I grieved the loss of my unborn daughter, and the vision of what I thought my family was going to look like. I grieved for the ability to give my son a sibling. But more than anything, I grieved for the person I was before I had endured so much loss. And when that part of me was spent, the anger took over, as it often does for people who have experienced such immense grief.

As the aftermath of months ticked on, I became very clear on what I was angry about. I was angry that this had happened to me. Especially after everything I'd already lost. I was angry that I was forced to make a decision I didn't want to make; just as I was learning to let go of control with my miscarriages, God flipped the script on me. I was angry that I was responsible for ending my unborn child's life; I was furious that God made me sit in the driver's seat for that one. I was angry that my husband seemed to move on from it much quicker than I did—I felt so alone in all of it. It took several years, months of marriage and grief counseling, and a lot of soul-searching to finally learn how to swim in my ocean of grief and find my way to the surface where I could breathe.

My pregnancy losses will always be a part of me, but they no longer consume me. I've made my peace with that part of my journey, as well as with God. I'm not angry about it anymore. I think that I was given my journey for a purpose. I believe God allowed me to walk this path because He knew I'd have the strength and courage to share it with others.

Over the past few years, I've openly shared my experiences with miscarriages and abortion with my friends and clients, as well as via social media. The overwhelming love and support I received played a huge part in my healing process. Pregnancy loss, abortion, and fertility struggles are so common, yet so many women are forced to struggle silently because they don't know who to talk to. Opening up about my experiences has allowed me to connect with so many women, and allowed me to create a safe space for them to share their experiences and struggles with me; this allows both of us to continue on in our healing process.

At the very least, I know I can give the gift of momentary solace, so these women who are truly suffering—they know that they're not alone. I have worked hard to find that silver lining in my story. Stories like mine don't always have a seemingly happy ending. But amid the messiness and heartbreak, I have found meaning, purpose, and so much joy.

I don't look at my story as one of loss. Though loss is a part of it, it's a story about life and love—having my son is the heart of my story. He was, and is, my greatest blessing. He gave greater meaning to my life, despite how much loss I endured. The loss has only amplified my gratitude for the blessings I've received in my life, especially Camden. Eventually I was able to embrace my grief, as it will forever be a part of me. I realized that grief and love go hand in hand. Without the grief, I never would've experienced the deep love God briefly blessed me with during each of my pregnancies. Love quietly lives in the empty space of each of my losses, which I will carry with me forever.

I chose to stop grieving all that I lost, and all that could've been, so that I could focus on loving the life that I have. Because it's a vibrant, beautiful life.

~ For Camden and my angel babies ~

Sarah Goldsborough is a boy mom to an amazing seven year old, Camden. He is her miracle rainbow baby, and her inspiration for sharing her journey. Sarah is a well known hairstylist in the Baltimore area, where she lives with her husband Larry, and son Camden. She prides herself on being somewhat of an open book, and has connected with many of her clients and friends, also dealing with pregnancy losses. She has shared her experiences and journey via social media as well, and has found it to be a big part of her healing process. Sarah loves to find humor in all things, and believes that laughter is the best medicine. You can follow her on Instagram @mommyyousaidthefword and @sarahgoldsborough

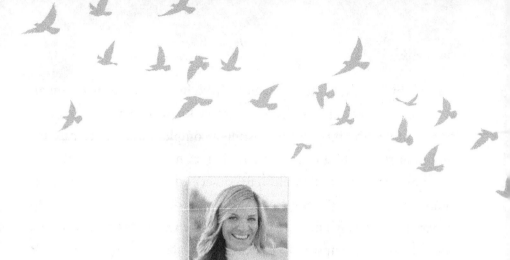

THE ONLY WAY OUT
IS THROUGH

Amanda Phoebus

I pray that we can find someone to help us carry our child who shares a similar perspective on surrogacy as we do and that we can change lives together by sharing our story. I pray that our future surrogate feels how hard we love in our family and that we will treat her no differently. I pray that she knows how much she will change our lives and how we feel grateful for her prior to ever meeting her. I pray that our children will see a different way to build a family and feel the love and respect that we have for one another. I pray that our surrogate feels supported, loved, respected, and appreciated wherever she is in her world right now. Thank you for following your own heart which has led you to this place, and we can't wait to meet you.

(Excerpt from my letter to our surrogate mother, 2021)

I never in a million lifetimes could have imagined another woman carrying my baby. In fact, I never even knew something like that was possible! The thought of trusting a complete stranger to care for and nourish *my* child inside *their* body for an entire nine months? At one point in my life, I would have described that as a form of cruel punishment, for everyone involved. Some other woman getting to experience my baby's first kicks and be woken up in the middle of the night by little hiccups, not to mention the actual birth of my child? Rip my heart out, why don't you!

It is funny how life teaches us, time and time again, that some of our preconceived notions about what we are afraid of or what we are sure "we would never do" are just made-up beliefs with no objective evidence to support them. After years of trying to give our daughter a sibling, I was faced with the reality that my only option to have another genetic child would be to do so via gestational carrier (surrogate). Suddenly, something that I once would have described as a form of torture or as my worst fear was *nothing* in comparison to my fear of simply not being able to have another child of my own. But if I were to explore even more deeply, when I broke it all down, I realized what I was terrified of was not having a sibling for my daughter. How this baby arrived into our lives did not matter as much as I had once believed. The only thing that mattered was that our baby would come to us healthy and that our daughter would not grow up an only child like I had.

I never had a chance at a normal childhood. Somewhere around age four, I would recognize this as my mom and dad screamed at each other in the kitchen a few rooms away. I vividly remember sitting in our den, getting lost in books like *The Very Hungry Caterpillar* and *Madeline*, pretending I was inside the story, away from my own home and what was happening in it. As I turned each cardstock page to discover what the caterpillar had eaten next, the angry screaming would grow louder, and looking back, what should have been a quiet, calm, and nurturing bedtime routine was often replaced by me crawling into bed by myself and falling asleep to the sound of my parents fighting. It seemed like they could get violent, but never quite did, and even at four years old, I knew something wasn't right about this.

As an only child in this type of home, I quickly learned that my "hunches" were accurate; things were not right. My mother was born with schizoaffective disorder, which is a devastating mental illness that combines schizophrenia with depression and bipolar disorder. My maternal grandfather had schizophrenia, which was much more life-altering and debilitating, but neither would I wish on my worst enemy. My mother's illness was managed by medication, but like many mental illnesses, without consistency in meds and doctors, the effects of the disease are immense. My father was a Vietnam veteran with a drinking problem and a lot of anger issues he never addressed. When the two of them were together, it was like we were in the middle of a volcano on the verge of eruption. Individually, both of my parents had enormously pure hearts. There is truly nothing negative I can say about them as humans, but unfortunately, they were each dealt cards throughout their lives that made it difficult for them to create a stable home for a child. This is what motivated me so profoundly to change my fate.

As a child, I was left to figure out much of life on my own. By the time I was five years old, my parents had separated. My mother and I moved in with my maternal grandmother and her second husband— Nana and Poppop. Nana and Poppop would be a tremendous force of stability during my childhood, teaching me how to cook, clean, make my bed, brush my teeth, garden, decorate the house for holidays, and so much more. I attribute a lot of my homemaking skills to the time I spent with Nana specifically, as she cooked every meal from scratch and would ensure I finished every last bite of my vegetables.

After living with them for a year, my mom secured a small apartment in the suburbs of Philadelphia, so we moved out. The apartment had two bedrooms, a tiny kitchen, an even tinier bathroom, and a living room. It was small, but it was ours. I took a lot of pride in keeping our apartment tidy and cozy because it made me feel safe in an otherwise unstable environment. My mom could only hold jobs for a few months, so money was tight, and most of our income would come from monthly social security checks. We bought food with stamps and received boxes filled with Hamburger Helper and ramen noodles from our church. My mom had a habit of opening credit cards, maxing out the limit, and starting the process over again. As a young child, I did not understand the responsibility that came with a credit card, so each time she opened a new account, it felt like Christmas morning just knowing that we could go to the grocery store and fill our cart with the same foods all the other families did. Most kids would beg for toys or candy when given the option of getting a treat, all I ever wanted was a pantry full of OREOS and Cheerios and a refrigerator full of food. I longed so deeply to feel normal.

Growing up with a mother who had a mental illness was much like growing up without a mother at all. So many moments were ruined when she could not discern reality from paranoia, right from wrong, or emotion from logic. Simple moments like getting ready for school in the morning or for bed at night became unnecessarily challenging and volatile. I was being raised by someone that was constantly having disordered thoughts and could offer very little guidance on typical adolescent issues such as friendships, school, and life. Throughout my childhood, my desire to be "normal" continued to grow. I often felt lonely, and it was part of what would drive me to do well in school, join sports teams, become part of the band and choir, and any other extracurricular group that would have me. Spending time with friends and their families was my survival guide—the more I surrounded myself with examples of stability, the more I learned how to create a stable life for myself. People were aware of my home life, but I became skilled at hiding the worst parts. I would go to great lengths to fake it was all normal at home, in front of friends, their parents, teachers—to the point that telling lies about my home life was a better option than ever letting on the truth.

Despite all of this, I still loved my mom. I knew that life did not have to look like this, and it was somewhere between ages five and ten that I started to identify with being extremely independent. Although I often felt alone, there was a constant knowing in me that if I stayed positive and worked hard in whatever I did, I could change my life. This "knowing" I would later realize was my intuition, guiding me through the highs and lows. It kept me grounded, it kept me hustling, and it gave me hope.

As I got older this practice of normalizing my abnormal stuck with me, but in a much healthier way. Over time, I became more comfortable sharing the realities of my family and my childhood. I found it was easier to be honest about my home life when I was removed from it during college. It was during this time that I started the long process of healing through therapy, and through that, I became comfortable sharing what growing up had been like for me. College was also the time that I started to realize how close my peers were with their families—making plans to go home for weekends and holidays to celebrate traditions and spend time with siblings and parents. I was very close with my dad by this point in my life, and while we would spend holidays together and it was incredibly special, I always wished we were a bigger family with lots of people and laughter and memories to make. A sense of longing started to develop for me, and that time in my life really changed the way I felt about what I wanted my future to look like. I felt just as strongly about creating a large family as I did about building a successful career, and as I neared the end of college I was feeling more confident than ever in my ability to have both.

To my absolute shock, two weeks before I graduated college, my dad suddenly passed away from a heart attack. His death robbed me of the only parent I had ever been able to lean on, solidifying that I was officially on my own. I was left to plan his funeral, take over all of his finances, rental properties and bills, by myself—all at the age of twenty-three. Losing my dad propelled my beliefs about what I hoped my family would look like one day. I would never wish being an only child on anyone when dealing with a parent's death, no matter what age.

The years after my college graduation were entirely devoted to advancing my career. I was driven like no other, singularly focused on attaining financial independence and forging a new path for myself. Through hard work, I climbed the career ladder, landing promotions that led to a level of financial stability I had never known growing up. Meeting my husband through work added another layer of fulfillment to my life, and after three years of dating, we tied the knot in 2015. Brian was the oldest of four, with three younger sisters, two of which had multiple children already. During our dating years, I was quickly launched into what life was like as part of a large family. The bustling holidays I had always dreamed of came to life and became a reality for me. There was so much about our new life together that answered many unspoken prayers for me, and to my greatest surprise, after less than a year of being married, we became pregnant with our daughter Lucy.

Nervous and excited, I lived the dream I had always envisioned. Our daughter arrived in Baltimore, Maryland, on March 23, 2017, marking the beginning of a year that felt like a fairy tale. Navigating life in the city with a newborn brought challenges and moments of pure joy, and as we settled into our new routines, I didn't think much about trying for another child. Lucy was conceived so easily, and the pregnancy was smooth. We assumed the second time around would be similar.

To understand how we arrived at our surrogacy journey, I must first explain Lucy's birth story as the two are forever intertwined. I went into labor four days prior to my due date and ended up having an extremely difficult delivery. My contractions started at 10:00 p.m., and after seven hours of intense pushing (and an epidural that did not work), a labor that I fully expected to be a walk in the park because of my age and athleticism turned into one of the biggest mountains I would ever climb. Lucy was progressing to the point where every doctor in the room commented "Look at that head of hair!!" At first, the comments about her hair helped to calm me, knowing that if they could see her hair, that meant we were making progress, and this pain would come to an end soon. But after the fourth or fifth person mentioned her hair, it occurred to me that she was in the same position and any progress I felt we had made, quickly dissipated.

Before 6:00 a.m. things took a turn when Lucy became stuck in the birth canal and subsequently lodged between my pubic bone and bladder. My hunch had been correct; she had not progressed and before I knew it, doctors were telling us we needed to rush to an emergency C-section. By this point, my body was so exhausted from pushing for the last eight hours I could barely muster any energy to ask questions about what was happening. The contractions kept coming, and I knew I needed to stay strong. The laboring process had sent Lucy and I into enough of a downward spiral that both of our vitals were plummeting. Simultaneously, doctors could see that Lucy had passed meconium which meant she was in fetal distress. One of my last memories before they wheeled me down long hallways to the OR was of me writhing in pain from the strongest contractions and zero epidural.

The OR was the brightest and coldest room I had ever been in; combined with the tense energy and quick moving doctors, I welcomed the sweet relief of anesthesia. Just numb enough to cut me open, they assured me I would be awake for the delivery. I was lying on the table for many minutes, cognitively aware that I had been cut open and then sensing a tremendous release from my abdomen. I knew Lucy was outside me, but the silence in the room brought on a form of panic I had never experienced in all my life.

"Why isn't she crying?" I asked my husband who was dutifully standing by my side. As my first feelings of motherhood angst washed over me, he assured me she was okay. Later, he would confess he felt less than assured by what he saw, but he was trying to keep me calm.

When the doctors pulled Lucy from my body, she was gray-faced and not breathing. They rushed her over to a table to pump the fluid out of her lungs and by the grace of God, within a minute, we heard her cry for the first time. She was brought over to me for a quick moment to say hello and then was rushed to the NICU to continue being monitored. I would remain on that operating table for over two and a half hours with no real understanding as to why. Brian would later describe this as the most terrifying hours of his life. He, too, was struck with a different type of panic as he watched doctors remove several organs from my body in search of the source of bleeding that they could not stop. In addition to the labor and delivery team, a urology team was called in, and I was surrounded by over ten doctors and nurses. Everyone in the room was afraid. I began vomiting, and in between retching, begged Brian to assure me everything was okay with our baby. After several hours of uncertainty, it was determined that the bleeding was caused by lacerations on my bladder that were a result of Lucy getting stuck during the labor process.

I was not allowed to hold Lucy during this traumatic experience, so after all my internal organs were replaced in my body, I spent the day waiting and praying that she was okay. Our prayers were answered when Lucy was returned to me the next morning—she was perfect! She was completely healthy and the largest baby in the NICU by far at 7 lb., 13 oz. My recovery was quick, and while the nightmare delivery was over and behind us, it would remain with us for years to come.

Our miracle daughter grew into the most beautiful gift I could ever have imagined. She has the heart of an angel, is full of light, and has brought so much happiness into our lives. We started trying for our second child when Lucy was over one year old. I did not feel a strong sense of urgency but decided to try sooner rather than later. I found it strange that after six months, we still weren't pregnant, and it didn't take long for my intuition to kick in that something was wrong.

In November 2018, we met with a fertility doctor for the first time and he quickly discovered that my entire uterus was covered in scar tissue. It was damaged so severely that it had completely lost its shape, and tests showed that there were serious concerns about the overall health and functionality of my uterus and its ability to carry another pregnancy. I was diagnosed with Asherman's syndrome, which essentially translated to scar tissue of the uterus. I spent hours, days, and nights researching cases of Asherman's syndrome, exposing myself to both the horrors and successes of this syndrome, and then eventually losing myself in the what ifs.

Three months after our initial fertility appointment, I underwent my first surgery. The objective was to remove the scar tissue from my uterus so that I could get pregnant again. I had a hysteroscopy done, as well as a laparoscopy, procedures that allowed doctors to access my uterus from different angles and attempt to clear the scar tissue. The immediate results provided grim feedback from my doctors. My surgeon explained that my uterus had been badly scarred. While he was able to clear the scar tissue, the scarring had changed the shape of my uterus so much that it had completely collapsed in some areas. The prognosis was simple: my uterus wasn't as healthy as before my labor with Lucy, and the scar tissue was likely to grow back again.

On our way home from this appointment, I couldn't stop crying. The one thing I had been dreaming of my entire life was being ripped away from me. The ability to have more children was the most important thing in my life; in that moment, it became crystal clear. As my mind struggled to process my reality and what this meant for our family, one word entered my mind: surrogacy. I didn't mention it to Brian as we made our way home, but the idea had come from somewhere deep inside my soul and gave me what I needed in that moment: a glimmer of hope.

What initially sounded like something that could be fixed with surgery was later described as one of the worst cases my doctors had ever seen. Experts from all over the country were working on my case, and the quest to figure out how to "fix" my uterus became all-consuming. I traveled to Boston to have surgery with one of the best doctors in the country. I fully expected to leave his office with confirmation that I would not be able to carry again, but after he cleared the scar tissue, to my surprise, he told me that there was enough healthy lining in my uterus to make it possible to carry another pregnancy. After a few more months of hormones and a round of IVF, I was able to harvest six embryos; after a long year of waiting, we transferred our highest-graded embryo; almost a year after the process began, I felt great hope as we finally cleared the scar tissue. I was convinced that after nine months of treatment and surgeries, my uterus was ready to grow a baby. Ten days later, we experienced what would become the first of many devastating phone calls. They all started the same: "I'm so sorry, Amanda," and then after a long pause, "the embryo did not stick."

Soon after our failed embryo transfer, I went in for my third surgery to check on the scar tissue. I wasn't surprised to hear that some of it had grown back. The feedback from my doctors implied the existence of the scar tissue was the only thing that would prevent a pregnancy, so I did not hesitate to agree to surgery after surgery. However, around this time, I decided I needed to do some more serious advocacy for myself and stop blindly trusting everything the doctors were telling me. After multiple surgeries that did little to fix my uterus, and feeling like no one was doing anything differently or trying to think outside of the box, we decided to transfer our embryos to a new fertility clinic in hopes of a fresh start. We were optimistic we would meet the golden doctor with the answers we needed.

Our new clinic recommended a fresh round of IVF, another surgery, and an Endometrial Receptivity Analysis (ERA), which is a test used in reproductive medicine to assess the best timing for embryo transfer during IVF. I lived at the doctor's office; there were moments where I was tempted to ask them if I could just leave an overnight bag, I was there so much. Several months went by, due to unexpected delays because of COVID-19, and by the time the clinic opened back up again, I was anxious to try another transfer. Six months later, we transferred two embryos, both of which were highly graded. My hopes had never been higher. We had a new clinic, new protocol, two embryos, and a receptive lining—this was going to work. It had to.

Ten days later, our hearts were broken once again when we found out that neither of the embryos had implanted.

Absolutely crushed after this loss, devastated, angry, exhausted, and afraid, I just couldn't understand why this was happening to us. It had been almost two years of non-stop fertility treatment and endless loss. Our friends on similar fertility journeys had all become pregnant by this point—it felt like it was never going to happen for us.

Every single area of my life had taken a backseat to my fertility journey. I was a shell of myself in so many ways, and could not think about anything other than our last failure and our next steps. In some ways, obsessively thinking about what was next was therapeutic as it allowed me to focus on potential solutions rather than on stewing in what was broken. But because I was investing a significant amount of my time and energy into our journey, it left very little remaining for everything else. Lucy still took up the rest of what I had to offer, but when it came to my job, my friends, and even my husband—the pain of what we were going through was taking its toll.

I had been wanting another baby for so long, and after *years* of trying, had nothing to show for it other than an extra fifteen pounds and a few scars on my body. My friendships became challenging to navigate as many of my girlfriends were getting pregnant with their second and third children during this time. Informal chats at work became impossible as I did not have the energy to engage in small talk. I could no longer participate in casual catch-up conversations with friends and family because anything having to do with family planning or having babies was triggering for me. I found myself distancing myself from those around me that I did not feel could empathize with my situation, which felt like everyone. Nobody I knew had struggled for this long on their fertility journey—why us?

I was lonely, depressed, and extremely difficult to be married to.

We would realize years later, but during these dark days of our fertility journey, a tiny, almost unrecognizable, wedge started to develop between Brian and I. Nothing tangible occurred that we could look back and say when it happened, but we were two humans separately suffering, and desperately trying to be there for one another. Brian was certainly there for me more than I ever was for him—which was never my intention, but looking back it was a brutal reality. He was steady, supportive, and truly my rock. But nobody was there for him to lean on. Although not bearing the brunt of this journey from a physical standpoint, emotionally he was with me every step of the way. He watched as I would force feed myself pills, helped me poke my body with needles, carried me through the doors of every surgery, helped me to pray and keep faith when it was hard finding a reason to do so, only to watch it crumble over and over again with no end in sight. It was the elephant in the room that brought our once light and fun-loving lives to a screeching halt. For Brian, another child was something he always wanted, but after three years of hitting the same devastating wall over and over again, he started asking why. Why did I keep doing this to myself? Why was I putting myself through this seemingly never ending pain? What was this all for, and when is enough enough? Lucy was our miracle child, she was perfect (truly)—when could we close this chapter?

I'm not exactly sure when it happened, but at some point, I entered survival mode. It was a mode I knew well from my childhood, where independence runs so deeply through my veins that anyone or anything that tries to stand in between me and where I want to be evaporates into my dust. Lucy as an only child just was not an option. My brain had been wired by trauma to understand only one version of life as an only child, and the emotions and memories associated with this were so extremely painful, it was almost like I was living in the turmoil and agony of my own childhood again. I was fighting so hard to prevent Lucy from being an only child that I could not see the reality: because of the work I had done in my own life, Lucy's childhood would look entirely different from mine. But I was operating from my survival instincts and beyond logic at this point—I was operating from my own experiences and I felt nothing in my life had ever been worth fighting for more than this. Despite all of the pain, the knowing was always right there, just like it was when I was a little girl. There was a light at the end of this tunnel; I just needed to be strong enough to see my way through.

We spent the next several months in and out of the fertility clinic. I had my fifth hysteroscopy to check my uterus for new scar tissue, did another round of IVF to create new embryos that we could genetically test, and when I wasn't in the doctor's office, I was on the phone fighting with the insurance company about what they would cover, wanting explanations for what they wouldn't. I was utterly exhausted. But even more than exhausted, I was angry, I was devastated, and I was so afraid—tempted to throw in the towel and admit defeat. But I kept going.

After two and a half years, almost one thousand days, I had consistently been on some sort of prescription hormones, birth control, progesterone, and estrogen. My body had not felt like my own in so long. After a fresh round of IVF (that we paid for out of pocket) showed we had two normal embryos from a total of seven harvested, we did another ERA test to ensure my lining still looked good, and one week later, we transferred our best-graded euploid embryo. This was the fourth embryo we transferred over eighteen months, and once again, we did not get pregnant.

As I put the phone down after another "Amanda, I am so sorry" from the doctor's office, I knew this was the end for me. The immediate understanding I experienced in these moments following that dreaded phone call was a blinding yet clarifying light. I wanted a baby. Did it matter how our baby got here? As long as he or she was healthy and here? I knew the answer, I always had. I could have everything I ever wanted and not have to suffer any longer. I never believed that sentiment until this very moment, but I knew that we could have another genetic child of our own if I gave up control over how he or she got here. Surrogacy had always been waiting for us, we just needed to choose it.

Approximately ten minutes after finding out we were not pregnant, I sent a message over Instagram to a friend of a friend who had recently shared pictures of her baby shower for her second child who was being carried by a surrogate. We were on the phone less than an hour later, and she graciously answered all my questions. She was a stranger to me and willing to share her entire journey. She readily gave me tips and advice to start making calls to surrogacy agencies so we could find the right one for our situation. I consider her my first of many angels in the journey to pursue surrogacy. No sooner than hanging up the phone with her, I sent a message on Facebook to an agency I had been following and asked if we could set up an introductory call. Once again, within another hour, I was on the phone with the agency and asked my initial questions about the process, next steps, and other logistics.

What the hell am I doing? This is completely insane! I kept thinking as I jotted down the information being given to me by the clinic. But while my head couldn't understand what a trajectory like this could look like, my heart knew this was the way to go. In a matter of minutes, my mindset shifted from obsessively trying to fix my uterus to being motivated as hell to find a suitable surrogate for our family. As we contemplated going down this road, a sense of peace came over me for the first time since the nightmare had begun. I felt that I had full access to my heart in this moment, and despite the doctors still telling me that I could carry a pregnancy myself, I made a decision that, deep down, I felt was right. My intuition had never taken me in a wrong direction. Why would I stop trusting it now?

Things started falling into place once we made the decision. We quickly connected with a surrogacy agency and were given an expectation of six months to find a match for a surrogate. Within one month of signing on with our agency, we matched with a woman who would go on to carry our baby. For the first few weeks, once we matched, we weren't allowed to communicate directly, but once we were given the green light to text and call each other, it was almost like a love story had begun.

We matched with our surrogate based on each other's profiles detailing our family life, profession, and fertility journey. Still, it wasn't until we had a video call and delved into the reasons behind our respective situations that we truly felt a connection and decided to move forward. After that point, there were many steps to progress toward an embryo transfer. The steps would include a complete medical physical by my doctor to ensure she was fit to carry, legal paperwork on both sides, blood work for Brian and me as well as her and her husband, and an incredible amount of emotion. She and I would communicate daily, just to chat about our lives and where we were in the process. After several months of working through the logistics, we finally attempted our first transfer. After a few rounds of drugs to get our surrogate's lining ready for a transfer, we were disheartened to learn that her uterus was not responding to the medications. We had to cancel our first cycle and start fresh—a setback that could certainly have sent us into a spiral at this point in the process—but we were steadfast in our pursuit. It took another two months to get through the holidays and additional issues with her lining, but finally, after three and a half years leading up to this point, we were ready to transfer one of our remaining three embryos.

Ten days later, we found out we were not pregnant.

This time, I was not only dealing with my own heartbreak, I felt the heartbreak of the woman who had selflessly dedicated herself to this process in hopes of giving my family a miracle baby. This was even worse, as I felt an incredible amount of guilt that someone was going through such an agonizing physical and emotional experience on my behalf. I knew how difficult and all-consuming it was for me; I could only imagine how it affected her and her family. We discussed the possibility of finding another surrogate or going through another round of IVF due to the transfer not taking—we only had two embryos left. The thought of going through another IVF cycle was unimaginable for me at that point. Despite the circumstances, I knew I needed to trust my heart on next steps, and sticking with our surrogate felt so right. I came to terms with the fact that I needed to be in a place where I would feel no anger or resentment toward her if this next transfer did not take, and she needed to know that as well. I decided to call her and communicate one simple message: if she gave this another chance with our last two embryos, it would be our best shot at this working but I would never blame her if it did not work out the way we wanted it to. She agreed, and we proceeded. In March 2022, we transferred our final two embryos—two embryos that were a combination from our very first IVF retrieval in 2019, as well as the second retrieval we did in 2021.

The wait over those next ten days was excruciating. And then, we got the call. This time, the phone rang and it was from our surrogate and her husband over FaceTime. The test was positive. She held the stick up so we could see the plus sign. We all hollered in excitement, "We are pregnant! We are pregnant!" Although at this point in the journey there were still a million things that could go sideways, the knowing inside of me could not have been stronger: I knew this baby would make his or her way to us. And I knew this was exactly how he or she was always supposed to arrive.

In the midst of finding out we were pregnant via surrogate, I would be lying if I said there wasn't a part of me that wondered if I could still have done this myself. No doctor had told me otherwise, so I found myself seeking closure. In the midst of our journey, my family and I had moved to New Jersey from Baltimore and we were now closer to the top fertility clinic in the country, one that was known for a particular doctor who provided research to clinics nationwide, including the ones in Baltimore that I had been working with. I waited months to see this doctor, as I needed to know I had seen the best.

My fear and anxiety immediately returned the second I stepped into the clinic—it came rushing back over me like a tidal wave, but knowing that we were already pregnant gave me an unmistakable sense of calm throughout the process. They performed many of the same procedures and tests I had done in the past, and after a complete evaluation, the doctor confidently shared his findings and prognosis with my husband and me. We sat on a video call and listened to him explain that IF I were ever to become pregnant (which he advised would be incredibly difficult given the shape and functionality of my uterus) *it would be fatal for me and the baby.* Essentially, the stem cells that make up the lining of the uterus had been permanently damaged during Lucy's delivery. Stem cells play a crucial role in regenerating and repairing the lining of the uterus and help maintain the health of the uterus—but when they are damaged, they are damaged. At the time, the medical world was just coming out with stem cell infusions that could have offered a solution, but the bottom line was that I had a verifiable explanation as to why the last three years had been fruitless. Naturally, this was a lot to process. I was relieved. I was sad. I was angry. Why had no other doctor found this? How much time could we have saved? Would I have even believed the other doctors without going through all the pain and loss myself? Why did I feel like I always had to take the hard way? What did I need to prove? All these thoughts and more would flood my mind for days, weeks, and months. Ultimately, I was grateful. Here I was with answers, and I had another baby on the way; here I was on a surrogacy journey that only came about because I had the confidence to trust myself.

Nine months after we got the positive pregnancy test, Brady Thomas Phoebus made his way earthside on November 30, 2022. In many ways, I was able to be more present for his birth than I was for Lucy's. The trauma of Lucy's delivery never allowed me to soak in the joy of bringing her into the world; I was too busy fighting for both of our lives. Brady's birth was textbook. The surrogate's water broke at 2:00 a.m. and by 7:09 a.m. he was here and in my arms. Brian and I were able to be part of the entire experience, and we both watched in awe as he emerged into our universe. Just thinking back on that moment still gives me chills when I recall those first seconds together. When the nurse handed him to me, the umbilical cord still attached, our eyes met and I was forever his mother. Brian was able to cut the cord, and once Brady was cleaned up and weighed, he remained on my chest for over an hour in the delivery room. Years of suffering were instantly wiped away as I held him in my arms. It was the purest connection I have ever felt, and as I kissed the top of his newborn head my heart said what I had known all along: "Oh, there you are. This was all for you."

A few months into Brady's life, I was in a yoga class one morning, moving through a sequence of sun salutations when tears began streaming down my face, as they often do in yoga. I was reflecting on our fertility journey and as I remembered the hardest moments, questions like "Why did it have to be this way?" or "Why did my delivery have to go like that?" and even "What did I do to deserve that?" came up. I had sat with these questions before, with little movement toward the answers. But here, in this moment, a knowing of the truth came to me: without the delivery that caused damage to my uterus there would be no Lucy. Everything needed to happen the way it happened so that Lucy could be here with us. And without Lucy, there would be no Brady. And without my childhood, there would not have been the strength to endure what it took to bring them both into the world. Despite my past and all the brokenness that raised me, I could see that I had always had the answers within. Without this journey, there would not have been the lesson I needed to learn in this lifetime: the knowing is inside of me. And when I dive even further into the lesson, I understand that I don't need to experience pain to experience joy. What a gift to carry with me for the rest of my days here on this earth, what a treasure I can pass on to Lucy and Brady.

Sometimes, perhaps always, the only way out is through. And it was through that saved my life and gave Lucy and Brady theirs.

Meet Amanda Phoebus, a devoted mother, loving wife, dynamic saleswoman, passionate writer, and wellness enthusiast. By day, Amanda serves as the Senior Vice President of Sales at Amwins. However, her most cherished roles are those of a mom to her two miracle children— Lucy, age 7, and Brady, age 1—a supportive wife to her best friend and husband, Brian, and a fur mom to their adorable pup, Hudson.

Beyond her family life, Amanda is deeply committed to fitness and wellness. She constantly strives to uncover her fullest self while inspiring others to do the same. Whether running along the beach, practicing yoga and Pilates, or embarking on exciting hiking adventures, Amanda believes in the transformative power of movement to rejuvenate both the mind and body.

Residing by the beach in Manasquan, New Jersey, she finds tranquility and inspiration in nature's beauty, which offers her a sense of calm and creativity.

Amanda is also dedicated to sharing her personal journey through fertility challenges to support others facing similar difficulties. Her mission is to uplift and guide individuals through some of life's toughest moments, empowering them to discover their strength, resilience, and hope along the way. You can connect with Amanda on Instagram @doedoe23.

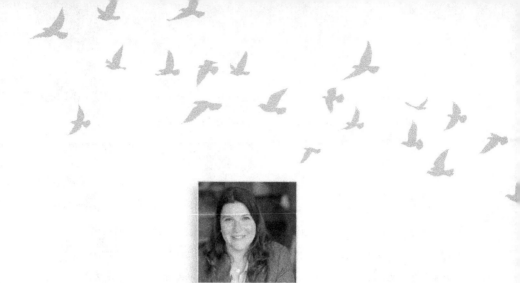

WHEN MEDICINE JUST ISN'T SMART ENOUGH

Sara Misconish Edwards

A good cry will crack your soul right open. Sitting on my favorite rock along the bank of the Cuyahoga River, I had the kind of cry that burst out of my body with brute force, against my tightly controlled will. The cry had been brewing for over a year, building day by day, pounding against the walls of my body begging to be let out. When my internal dam finally broke, a rush of emotions poured out of me, the tears releasing a tidal wave of painful failures from the last two years: six failed inseminations, dozens of pointless appointments, thousands of dollars spent, endless disappointment in my body, and fiery frustration at my experiences. I didn't know what I was getting into when we decided to start fertility treatment, and I didn't know if I wanted to go any further. It had been a long and arduous journey and, by all accounts, I was worse for wear. I felt like a failure, my marriage was strained, and I was crying alone in the woods. Something *had* to change.

A decade earlier, on a warm summer night in Cleveland, I rolled my old blue blanket out in the soft summer grass of my neighborhood park to enjoy a picnic and concert with my friends. Sitting cross legged, the sounds of latin jazz floating in the air, I was magnetically drawn to Bryan. We spent the evening playfully chatting and building our first inside jokes. In many ways, he was my opposite. I was a working artist; he worked in finance. I had spent the last decade assembling a chosen family; he had spent it sitting on the sofa with his grandma, watching *Dancing with the Stars.* As I was packing up to leave, we exchanged contact information and a jolt of electricity ran down my spine. *That's your person*, a voice whispered inside my head as I walked home. The very next morning, I sent him an email and we planned our first date for a few weeks later. I knew in my heart the voice was right.

After a few months of dating, we became inseparable. We liked being together so much that daily tasks like laundry and grocery shopping together became magical. On an ordinary Tuesday night, washing dishes after a homemade meal in my tiny apartment, the conversation drifted toward having our own family one day. Before Bryan, I was ambivalent toward motherhood, and at times, judgmental of it. I hadn't yet explored my indecision, but I found myself catapulted into a very serious conversation quickly. We had never discussed it before, and I could feel the nervousness associated with such a life changing topic rising in my chest as I stirred the peppers and onions and turned my eyes to the linoleum floor under my feet. *What if we didn't agree? Would he still be my person? What if he thought I was selfish for having mixed feelings?* We decided, instead of saying it outright, rather, we would write down a number that would measure how much we wanted a family on a scrap of paper. And then, we would switch. Bryan ran to grab a pad of yellow Post-its and some pens, and I took a deep breath. With my heart pounding and heat rising in my face, I took my tiny paper square and without much contemplation scribbled down a seven. A seven meant I was interested in it, but it was not the sole goal of my life. I could envision plenty of other futures that did or did not include kids, but I knew I wanted all of them to include Bryan. I quietly folded my square in half, and slid it across the table to him.

I waited nervously as Bryan slid his paper across the table to me. I looked him in the eye as I opened the paper slowly. Breaking our gaze, I looked down to see that right there, in his messy handwriting, was the number seven point five. I didn't realize I was holding my breath until I saw it. I exhaled out a huge sigh of relief at the match. Smiling at each other across the table, we started envisioning our future family together. *A baby boy, no, a baby girl*, with Bryan's eyes. She'd have my curiosity, he said, and I wanted his sense of humor for her. She'd be funny and smart, and love the outdoors. Somewhere, in the distant future, we were going to have a family. Decision made.

Shortly after we got married, we decided it was time to start our family. After being together for six years, well into our midthirties, we felt ready for parenthood. We had grown tired of the decadent joys of early adulthood and wanted a different kind of late night, one spent right here in our pale-yellow suburban home. When we decided that parenthood was in our shared future, we thought the hard part was making the decision. Looking back, it's almost cute how naive I was.

A year later, I find myself sitting in an unremarkable examination room, seeking answers from the oracle of modern medicine. I came here for answers, because I have a whole lot of questions. As The Doctor rattles off a slew of clinical terms I am desperately trying to make meaning of, I slowly come to understand that the mechanics of my body are broken in a way that couldn't be understood, even by her. A year of failed attempts at pregnancy awards me the official diagnosis of "unexplained infertility." While The Doctor continues to speak, I realize the truth of the message: *there are no answers.* There is nothing to fix because they can't identify what is wrong. They explain to us that parenthood is possible, but will require medical intervention. I feel my presence leave the conversation and tunnel deep inside my thoughts. *Infertility? What do they mean by unexplained? Does that mean I can never have a baby? What caused this? Why did this happen to me?* I leave with a ten-page treatment plan, a long list of supplements that are meant to support a deficiency that can't be defined, and suggested lifestyle modifications that bring on an overwhelming sense of doom.

The paperwork sits on our dining room table for a week before I can talk about it. I don't want to acknowledge it. Somewhere inside I believe that avoiding it will make the diagnosis less true. It's overwhelming to have a physical condition that is both concrete and ambiguous—*yes, you are infertile but exactly why, we do not know.* And because they don't know, they aren't sure how to fix it. Questions swirl through my head: *What exactly am I inviting into my life? How much effort will it take to get pregnant? Will it be painful? Will this turn our sex life into work? What will this do to our relationship? What happens if it doesn't work?* These are the questions that swirl in my head, filling the air between us at dinner each night, as the paperwork sits, an uninvited guest at the head of the table.

We made a plan to discuss it over steaming hot pancakes at a neighborhood breakfast joint, our favorite spot for serious conversations. Sipping the bitter diner coffee, Bryan makes his case for moving forward with medical intervention. From his perspective, we don't know what's wrong, so we have little ability to change the outcome on our own. We watched friends struggle and we saw the way it wore them down. We bought our home in a family-friendly neighborhood because a family was what we wanted, right? My points were grounded in protecting myself. I wasn't sure what the interventions would entail, but I knew they wouldn't be pleasant. I was also dubious of an unexplained condition with a concrete intervention. If they didn't know what was wrong, how could they be so sure this would work? As we pored over the decision from every angle, we decided that trying it once couldn't hurt. After all, if it was effective, we would have nothing to worry about.

We decide to take another step down the path of parenthood and say yes to medicine's help. Our plan is to have an intrauterine insemination, colloquially known as an IUI. Before we can even get to the procedure, we have to tackle the massive to-do list they gave us: five daily supplements, a Clomid prescription, and pages of diet and lifestyle modifications.

The Doctor did not prescribe hypervigilance, but that quickly became my default mode of operating. Despite my ambivalence towards motherhood, I am resentful that the choice was snatched away from me unexpectedly. Infertility activated tendencies I didn't love about myself: my desire to control, a laser focus on achievement, the urge to meet the expectations of others, and putting myself dead last on the priority list. It excavated every insecurity and played them on repeat in my head. I wanted to uncover why this was happening, and in the absence of any reason, I blamed myself. *Was this my fault? Was I selfish? Had I waited too long?* At the best of times, these thoughts whispered to me in silent moments. At their worst, they became paralyzing, blocking all other thoughts out.

I began to look for anything to change my circumstances to feel a small semblance of control. I obsessively tracked my biometrics with the precision of a research scientist. Every morning, I set the alarm and scheduled my first pee so the fertility strip data was consistent. After that I took my temperature and added it to my log. I stripped gluten from my diet and ate vegetarian. I threw out any reusable plastic and replaced it with glass, in case it contained endocrine disruptors. I quit drinking alcohol and watched my social life shrink. Optimizing my fertility was not just a hobby, it was my new part-time job and it consumed me. I sincerely believed that if I did everything perfectly, we would find ourselves pregnant in no time.

When the fertility strip reveals it's IUI go time, Bryan leaves for his appointment first, and I leave for mine shortly after. Craving support from each other, we're sad to learn our appointments are in different locations and separate us when we're already vulnerable. When I nervously walk into the clinic for the first time, it becomes painfully obvious that we are now part of a new club: the Secret Society of Hopeful Parents. I immediately resent my membership to this club—it, in fact, was not consensual. But as I look around, I realize no one wants to be here. We all anxiously scroll on our phones and avoid eye contact, waiting for our appointment to come so we can get out of there as quickly as possible. When the receptionist slides open the window and calls my name, I spring to my feet and slink over to her, doing my best to be invisible.

"That'll be $742," she says flatly, with a hint of disdain.

"I'm sorry, what did you say?" I stammer back. I'm not expecting to have to pay anything other than a co-pay on the day of the procedure.

"It's $742 for the procedure." She looks past me to the other patients taking up space in the waiting room.

"Can you bill me?" I ask weakly.

The receptionist shook her head as her gaze went from behind me to meet my face. "No, we need to collect payment before you go back to see the nurse since this is a self-pay procedure and not covered under insurance." Ah, there it is.

Despite our hushed tones, her clipped behavior leads me to sense I'm making a scene. I fumble through my purse and fish out my credit card. Slide, swipe, sign, and the price of entry is paid. A hefty fee for a club I didn't want to join. I quickly go back to the chair I had been occupying and sit back down to await my turn. Every cell in my body wants this to be over.

For all the effort leading up to it, the actual appointment is short and transactional. I undress from the waist down, crawl onto the exam table, place my stocking feet into the stirrups, and stare into the square fluorescent lights until I see the inverse image behind my closed eyes. The nurse slides her stool over and thrusts a vial of sperm way too close to my face, confirming that it is, indeed, the product of my partner, birthdate 1982. I nod quietly as panic, revulsion, and fear travel from my stomach and settle into a knot in the back of my throat. I focus my mind back on the ceiling, counting the tiles, and running little math problems in my brain to distract myself. *8 x 9 = 72.* As hard as I try to get lost in the calculations, the rustling of medical supply packaging brings my focus back to her. Anxiously scanning the walls, I spot a clock and notice how slowly the seconds tick. The nurse announces she's ready, and I watch the minute pass second by second. She was in and out of my uterus in under thirty seconds, throwing the used catheter into the biohazard bin and whipping open the door to leave. She brusquely states the discharge instructions as she walks out: "Keep your feet in the stirrups for the next ten minutes, then leave."

Flustered and alone, I noticed the nervous sweat cooling on my forehead, making the chilly room feel colder. I wanted something comforting, like a blanket or some gentle music while I waited. Instead, I passed the time shivering on the crinkly exam table paper and listening to the muffled conversations outside. When it's finally time to go, I stand up and look down at my abdomen with hope. *It's over,* I think to myself. Rubbing my stomach gently, I imagine it carrying our baby. I made it through the checklist, endured the nurse's hostility, and expected my A+ efforts to pay off. On my way out I pause to look back at the room, and think, *At least I'll never have to come back here.* I stroll down the hall and meet Bryan in the parking lot, envisioning our joy at a positive pregnancy test.

Two weeks later, I was genuinely surprised when I woke up to the start of my cycle. Dumbfounded, I went back to my list. I had done everything right, so what happened? When we decided to take this step, it felt like a sure thing. *How could it have failed? How could I have failed? What did I do wrong?* Self-blame settled in as I rifled through the bathroom cabinet for a tampon.

I call to discuss next steps and learn The Doctor has left the practice. What's more, they won't tell me where she went. "We can refer you to another doctor," they offer. "However, there is a six month wait for an appointment."

Out of options, I put myself on the waitlist, hang up the phone, and scream *"ffffffuuuuuuuuuuuccccckkkkkkkk!"* at the top of my lungs into the empty kitchen. Sliding down the wall and falling to a heap onto the tiled floor, I'm shaking with rage. We waited months to see The Doctor, for this one important and very expensive appointment. Tears stream down my face as I realize the reality: I have absolutely no control.

A few weeks later, Bryan and I discussed second opinions, but after an antagonistic entry into fertility medicine, I'm hesitant. I felt like an object by the gruff staff and disappearing doctor. Holding hope for both of us, Bryan doesn't see the harm in talking to them. *That's easy for you to say. It's not your body on the table*, my subconscious whispers. Still, I push my discomfort aside and make an appointment with The Hospital for a second opinion in a few weeks.

We go to the appointment together, and it immediately feels different. The receptionist rolls open the window and welcomes us to the office with a smile. She doesn't rush us, but rather, makes small talk as I go through the extensive list of first-appointment patient forms. The walls are covered in their own sort of wallpaper, hundreds of birth announcements for babies they played a part in creating. When our name is called, we are greeted warmly by a smiling nurse. The Physician's office feels academic but not stuffy. A large mahogany desk covered with books and research studies anchors the room. We take our places in the two velvet chairs that face the desk and make room for our low expectations to settle in with us.

The Physician shares that he has helped many couples "like us" become parents. "Unexplained infertility just means medicine isn't smart enough to understand why you haven't been able to get pregnant. Eventually

137

we will learn, but we don't know . . . yet," he matter of factly states. I find his crisp acknowledgement of my experience and medicine's role in failing us refreshing and hopeful to hear. This isn't my fault and success isn't up to me or a result of my actions. Despite a lack of insurance coverage, this is a real health condition that should be treated like a chronic condition, because I feel real, consistent, long-term impacts. My body releases the tension it's been carrying for months and I sink into the chair giving full trust to The Physician. He recommends we continue with the treatment plan. If we're not pregnant after six IUIs, we can discuss in vitro fertilization—IVF. We leave feeling seen and supported, genuinely optimistic that our outcome will change. We head to our favorite diner, this time celebrating the twist of fate that turned an MIA doctor into a hopeful second opinion. We raise our coffee mugs and toast to our good fortune and the future we could envision again.

Within six weeks, we were back in the velvet chairs after another failed IUI. The swell of hope retreated as quickly as a wave at low tide. We churned through March, April, May, and June at a swift pace, just to find ourselves with four more failures. Each month took us back to the beginning, with lighter pockets and dwindling hope. The biometric data in my spreadsheet no longer felt like an equation I could solve. It felt futile. As much as I tried to control and reconfigure the inputs, the output remained the same: not pregnant. I was trapped in a paradox of monitoring my body with precision but feeling increasingly disconnected from it. To get through each day, I imagined myself tucking all of my feelings in a black shoebox, closing it tightly, and pushing it to the very back of my closet. *I'll deal with that later,* I thought to myself, but each week came and went and the box remained.

It became harder to share disappointing news with our family and friends each month. With every failed procedure, you could see the hope drain from their faces. I watched them search for comforting words: *Everything happens for a reason,* or, *It'll happen when you least expect it.* I knew they meant well, but each time someone offered "help," I felt rage flush through me. It became harder and harder for me to hold my tongue when responding. "What's the reason for an unexplained health condition?!" I once bit back. Every twenty-eight days, my cycle begins with disappointing predictability and my anger grows. With no place for the anger to go, I retreated into myself and shared less. I threw myself into my job, where I was competent, capable, and the spreadsheets always made sense.

Coming home from a long day at work, I walk into the living room, drop my work bag by the couch, and feel the electricity in the air. It's literally crackling. I can tell we're going to have THE conversation, or more accurately, THE fight that has been brewing for months.

"What we're doing isn't working," Bryan spats out in exasperation. We both know we need to consider IVF seriously. "Let's just try it once," he pleads with me. "If it were up to me, I would do it. I would do *anything* for us to have a family."

Exhausted and cornered, I lose my temper, more so at our predicament, rather than at him. "I don't want to go through that. This is my max. My body and my brain are tired." I let out an exhausted sigh. "I want to own my body again. I want to love it instead of despising it. I want to stop stressing it with medical instruments and pumping it full of hormones. I feel like you blame me, like it's all my body's fault, and that makes me hate it more." Suddenly I'm shouting these words, releasing the pressure of the last six months through a frenzy of omissions and accusations that flow down my sad face in fiery, furious tears. "I miss being friends and partners. I miss waking up with you and spending a carefree day together. Now, I wake up with the weight of infertility every day, knowing that I'm disappointing you and that it's possible the rest of our life together will be a disappointment. I wake up in the middle of the night, choking on panic that you'll leave me and choose another life where you can be a dad, because the one we have together isn't the one you want." I sob out my truth before I can change my mind. I look up from my hands and watch his face fall. I took this argument to another level.

"Oh, Sare, I'm so sorry," he says, tears threatening to break his voice. "I didn't know you were feeling that way. It's not your fault. I would never want to put that responsibility on you. I just feel so helpless and anxious and IVF seems like it would give us a better chance." His voice grew softer and he hesitated, but finally got the words out. "Would you at least consider exploring it?"

The fight dragged both of our positions out into the light: I didn't want to continue with fertility treatment, and Bryan wanted to up the ante. We decided we needed a break from all this and took a last-minute vacation to Banff, hoping to find peace and perspective in the Canadian Rockies. While glancing at beautiful turquoise mountain lakes, my mind was elsewhere and fearful thoughts churned in my brain: *Of course he wants to do IVF. He doesn't have to DO anything. I do. This would drain our savings. All he wants is a pregnancy. What happens to us if I say no? Will we survive? What if we get divorced? What kind of life would I have?* I hoped that a week in nature would open me to the possibility of IVF, but internally, I hardened into my no. I told Bryan I was open to learning about it, but we both knew it was half-hearted. After the trip, we called and scheduled the consultation. With a date months into the future, I was grateful for the reprieve from the fertility stress. *Were we willing to undergo more procedures and shell out thousands of dollars to become parents?* I had until March 19, 2020, to figure it out.

COVID-19 made the decision for us. A week after the World Health Organization declared a pandemic, we had our IVF consultation over Zoom, but it was pointless. The Hospital reassigned all clinicians to critical COVID patients and elective procedures like IVF were on hold indefinitely.

I was immediately relieved. I didn't realize how deeply I was resisting IVF until it wasn't an option. I hoped I would feel differently, but after months of poking and prodding I needed a break. I needed space to process the feelings I had been stuffing down to make it through another day, another appointment, another treatment. I had been in survival mode. The pause felt like a gift, giving us the ability to slow down and reconnect.

One April afternoon, after a long hike on my favorite trail, I walked to the river to sit on my "sad rock." Its smooth and sloped surface made it easy to sit cross-legged for longer periods of time and it became my favorite place to connect with my feelings. It was perched just above the waterline, as close to being in the river as you could get without getting wet. Peering into the water from the rock, I watched leaves travel down the river and get stuck in the spiraling eddy beside me. Like me, they were trapped by forces of nature beyond their control. Instead of fighting with all their might, they surrendered to the current and eventually spun out of the whirlpool and floated downstream. As I watched this pattern over and over again my internal monologue quieted down. Tears streamed down my face and dripped into the river when a courageous new voice emerged. *You have to let go*, it said. *The change that needs to happen is within you*, it whispered. I realized that in order to alleviate my pain, I had to acknowledge its existence and let it go.

I was finally brave enough to look at my situation for what it was: I had an unexplained medical condition that was changing the course of my life and threatening my marriage. Infertility had brought painful physical experiences but I was adding to my mental anguish. My coping strategies attempting to control it weren't working. Instead, they were breeding anger, fear, and sadness. I had plenty to infuriate me: the gaps in women's healthcare knowledge, the lack of insurance coverage, and the lack of cultural sensitivity to fertility issues made me seethe with rage and powerlessness. But the fear was deeply personal and cut to the bone. *What will happen to us if I can't have a baby? Is our relationship prepared to explore a new set of dreams beyond parenthood?* We deferred the "when will you have kids?" question from well-meaning family and friends for years. *What if the answer was* never? I sat on the sad rock for over an hour, letting the waves of feeling come and go, the cool spring air drying my tears.

By the time I returned home, I had been gone for hours. With one glance Bryan could tell something was bothering me. He guided me to the couch, brought me a hot cup of coffee, and asked me what was on my mind. Curled up on our old gray couch, tears welled in my eyes and everything came flooding out: the insights discovered on the sad rock, the pressure I felt to get pregnant, the sadness I had after so many failed attempts. We settled in for a conversation and examined every fear that unexplained infertility raised in us. I was afraid of disappointing him and fearful that each disappointment led us closer to losing our relationship. He was afraid that my fear of pain and loss would stop us from trying, and that keeping our sadness to ourselves would tear us apart. We talked until the sun went down, scrutinizing every what if that arose: *What if he wants this more than I do? What if I don't want to do IVF? What if we can't have our own child? What if our sadness and anger is too big for the other to hold?* Asking these questions was a bid for reassurance, for a recommitment to each other during this season of tribulation. Looking back, neither of us remembers the precise responses we gave to each other on the couch that day. What we do remember, is feeling safe enough to explore the uncertainty. In the end, the answers didn't matter. Sitting together with the unanswerable questions opened a portal of hope and strength for us both.

The next morning, we decided to put the infertility journey aside and make supportive choices for ourselves each day. I kept a little list of questions in my head to identify my needs: *How am I feeling? What do I need? What can I do to care for my body? What can I do to care for my heart?* Taking it day by day, we began to create rituals that nurtured stability and healing. We lovingly made coffee and green smoothies for each other every morning. We bought kayaks and took them out on Lake Erie as often as possible. We planted a little vegetable garden that we nicknamed "the farm," and as the little garden grew and eventually flourished, our spirits began to rebound too. As simple as it was, it felt good to take loving action toward my body and not force it through uncomfortable medical procedures. I was reconnecting with myself and discovering what I needed, which was a heavy dose of self-compassion. *Be gentle, be easy* became my guiding principle at the core of every choice as I slowly came back to myself over a deliberately languid summer.

One bright Sunday in early October, as we paddle our kayaks through a grove of trees, I decide it's the perfect opportunity to bring up the exciting topic of health insurance. Bryan squints at me and laughs, wondering if I really want to talk about health insurance here. After considering it for a few seconds, I decide, yes, I do. Fertility benefits are now offered by my employer and if we switch to my plan IVF will be covered. I share with him that I've thought about it, and I'm open to giving IVF a go, if it's available. His eyes widen with possibility, and he looks at me cautiously. "Really? You'd be open to trying it?" he asks carefully. I nod and smile as tears fill my eyes. Right there on the water, in a place that brings us so much healing, we gather our strength, resilience, and hope, and choose to begin again.

The next morning, I called The Hospital and learned IVF procedures would start in February 2021. I put myself on the waitlist and they would review our medical file in the meantime. Two days later, I received my IVF prep list: OB-GYN exam, a hysterosalpingography procedure, insurance pre-authorizations, and an enormous crate of drugs. I sigh heavily as I read through the tasks. Here we are again with another to-do list, but this time is different—because we are different. We've spent the last year healing the pain of our failed fertility treatments while surviving a pandemic. We're still here, while so many others aren't, and we can't help but come away from that with a wild sense of hope. We held each other closer, tended to our anger and sadness dutifully, and to our surprise, what could have been the breaking of us served as the fertile grounds of compassion and a deeper, stronger love.

We take it one day at a time and slowly complete each checklist item. Before each procedure, Bryan and I snuggle up on our old gray couch and make a plan for how we will care for each other. This time, there are absolutely no spreadsheets. We select rituals that ground us, like making our morning coffee together, taking walks, and watching nature documentaries. We start and end our days together as a team, checking in on how we feel and what we need. We decide to share only with the friends we know can sit with our experience and just listen. We bring in evidence-based care that supports the IVF process and feels relaxing, like acupuncture. If it doesn't follow our be gentle, be easy principle, then it's not for us, no questions asked.

We are lucky enough to have a successful egg retrieval and even luckier to have two embryos; one graded excellent and the other good enough. We choose to transfer the excellent embryo and steady ourselves for the long wait, bringing hope along for the ride. We lean into our rituals:

long hikes, elastic waist pants, and copious amounts of sleep. On the day of the pregnancy test, we take the day off from work and head to our favorite trail. Midhike, The Physician calls to deliver the news. The transfer failed and we need to try again. The trees feel like they're falling down on top of me, and I no longer hear what he is saying on the other end of the line. After I hang up, I realize we still have a long way to hike to get back to the car. With tears streaming down our faces, we spend the next hour hiking silently on our favorite path that will be forever tainted by the news. The next day, we pick ourselves up off the ground and call The Physician to strategize. He recommends another egg retrieval to create higher quality embryos than the one we still have to increase the odds of success. We take his recommendation and steel ourselves for another retrieval. We were so close this time, and we agree it feels right to try again.

Insurance doesn't agree with this strategy, and won't cover another retrieval while we have a frozen embryo. Yet again, we have no choice, and insurance calls the shots. It's a difficult decision to accept but at this moment, I'm at the will of insurance. Abiding be gentle, be easy means we take the easiest path forward, and today that means acknowledging how angry we are that insurance can change the course of treatment. On the flip side, we're grateful for insurance coverage that made this possible for us. Sitting with both feelings reminds us that the only thing we control is our response. We surrender to big insurance and prepare for another transfer.

We transfer our good-enough embryo, pushing the unfavorable conditions out of our mind and wait. When the pregnancy blood draw comes two weeks later, we take the day off and stay home; we learned our lesson last time and don't want another grief hike. We roam around the house with bated breath, trying to fill our hearts, minds, and hands with anything that will distract us. Laundry, gardening, and old episodes of *Girls* keep us busy. When the call finally comes, I let it ring twice before I pick up my phone, unsure if I want to learn what The Physician knows just yet. By some miracle, he says, this transfer worked. I was just over two weeks pregnant. Bryan dropped to the ground onto his knees, tears of gratitude rolling down his face as we listened to The Physician on speaker phone. It was finally happening, we were having a baby!

The next few weeks move by luxuriously slow as we keep our exciting secret. Given the ups and downs of the journey, we're hesitant to share the news until we're out of the first trimester, which is easy because we're still in a pandemic and social distancing. The people we do see have noticed a shift. They can't help but see our joy—it's radiant.

As my pregnancy progresses, I can't shake the fear of the unknown; this thought that at any minute, life can shift its course and change our plans and decimate our dreams. We've negotiated an uneasy peace with that fact and learned how to find agency in the ebb and flow. When I develop high blood pressure in the second trimester, I breathe and take it day by day. When we learn that the baby is breech at thirty-six weeks, we look at our options and choose what feels best for us. We opt for a version procedure, where OBs manually flip the baby by pressing on my uterus. With our delivery bags packed, we head to the hospital two weeks before our due date and expect to return home with a correctly positioned baby. While our baby flips like a little acrobat my already high blood pressure spikes, and we are admitted for an emergency induction, another unexpected wave to ride. After all, we have no choice.

It takes over seventy-three hours and twenty-two nurses, midwives, and clinicians to deliver our baby girl, but when she finally arrives everyone feels the miracle of her existence. There are too many people in the delivery room and they're all crying—the nurses, the midwife, and the resident, in awe of his first delivery. Bryan is stooped low and close, as near as he can be without crawling into the bed with me. We've spent over three days here together, and in the last hour I've ascended to an otherworldly realm. Every breath in and out of my lungs feels sacred. Tightly gripping Bryan's hand, I feel our hearts beating in sync. I can no longer tell where I end and he begins. The anger, pain, and sadness of the journey has alchemized into a powerful love for our new family of three. "I've been a midwife for fourteen years and I don't cry anymore at deliveries, but something about this one, and the way you two connect is special." Gazing lovingly at our moments-old daughter, her warm body on my chest, we tell her she has no idea how truly extraordinary this moment, this baby, this journey is.

Six years have passed since we first learned the term unexplained infertility, but its lessons are now part of our DNA. Infertility threatened everything I held dear: my marriage, our shared future, my sense of empowerment and strength. Those years are dominated by paradoxes. It was all consuming, but it gave us nothing. On the surface it appeared to be about a baby, but truthfully, it was about us. Obsessive control, punishing self-discipline, and repressing my feelings didn't bring me strength. They added to my pain. Instead, I found strength in facing the feelings that compelled me toward such forceful actions. Confronting the fear, anger, and sadness that infertility stirred up was my deepest act of courage. I didn't feel brave during the many days I spent crying on my sad rock, but the more I tended to my feelings, the less power they had over me. Each time, I walked away from the river gentler and stronger.

Everything ends, including infertility. It surprises me to say that I now see my experience as an invaluable gift. While I lost the version of me who started the journey, the new version lives with gentleness and compassion. I was lucky enough to walk away with a beautiful daughter, a stronger marriage, and a more loving perspective towards myself and the world. I'm no longer afraid of anger or sadness because they send us powerful messages we need to hear. If we're brave enough to listen, they reveal what matters, what's worth fighting for, and ultimately what we love. I'll never be the person I was before infertility, but now that I'm on the other side, I don't want to be.

Sara Misconish Edwards is a designer, strategist, and writer leveraging her talents to drive healthcare innovation. As the director of design operations at University Hospitals Ventures, Sara shapes the future of healthcare with a compassionate and humanistic approach. She also serves on the board of LAND studio, a public art organization. Sara resides in Shaker Heights, Ohio, with her husband and nature-loving daughter. To learn more about Sara connect with her on Instagram @HeySaraEdwards.

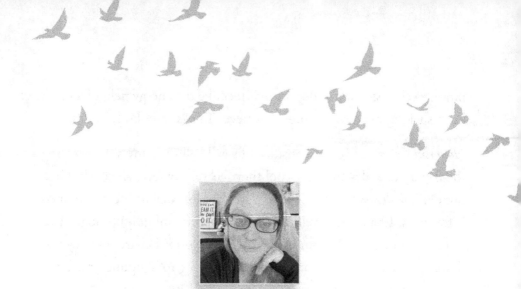

DEEP PAIN AND DEEP JOY—A COLLISION

Katie Jamieson

I've been here before. In this tiny four-by-five-foot bathroom, alone, confused, cold, in pain, nauseous, bleeding.

Shaking.

Katie, this is your fourth miscarriage. You should be better prepared for this. You know what to expect. You knew this one was coming for the past week: my gut instinct before the devastating ultrasound confirmed what I already knew. This wasn't viable. I have now been pregnant *six* times. None of this is new.

Except *this* is new. This loss and the way it's occurring. And the way I found out; at that Monday morning ultrasound the day after leading my biggest work event of the year. I feel devastation, grief, and an emotional illness swell inside me at depths that feel like the energy field of a black hole, sucking me down without reprieve. This is utter body betrayal.

How did I even get here? I consider this as I roll onto my side, noticing the frigid floor tiles and how cool they feel on my feverish cheek. I had done all the *should* things. I led the way. I had lost weight and maintained it for years. I had eaten well; exercised. I had (thankfully) brought two beautiful, healthy, full-term babies into the world. I charted my cycles, drank green tea, took supplements, and went to acupuncture. I got on progesterone as soon as I saw a positive pregnancy test. And as if those things weren't enough, I advocated for myself in every direction, tirelessly.

Despite the lived experience, the reality of what I am facing is too much.

You can't plan your way out of a miscarriage. And I was used to planning my way out of, around, and through . . . everything.

I don't know how much time I've spent in the bathroom, sometimes lying on the floor between painful clots and tissue-passing moments; other times, my body pressing against the door. At some point, I realize I'm rapidly dehydrating. I text my sister. She immediately calls me. "Katie. Put down the water and get Gatorade or you will have to go to the ER."

Anything but that. Being my fourth miscarriage, I know: avoid the ER. And I'd successfully done so the previous weekend, even though I have Rh-negative blood and need a RhoGAM shot with *any* bleeding I experience during pregnancy or miscarriage. I've had so many of these enormous needle shots in my hip at this point—it's unpleasant, and without it, my body could attack future pregnancies if the baby has Rh-positive blood. After failing to get help at an urgent care *and* an urgency room, an on-call doctor confirmed I could wait closer to the maximum of seventy-two hours from the start of bleeding. Thank goodness.

This time, I would manage to avoid the ER and instead visit the clinic Monday morning, only to end up with a loud, pushy, can't-read-the-room nurse attending me. "Well, this *is* a nurse visit, so we need your weight, and your blood pressure, and . . ."

"I've been through this before, and you don't need weight or blood pressure to give me a shot. Please give me the shot so I can leave." *Not my first rodeo, Nurse Dense.*

Taking a break from the cold bathroom floor, I sit on the bathtub's edge. My experience with the three previous miscarriages and pregnancy-related illnesses kicks in: *hydrate. Stay hydrated, Katie, and you can avoid the ER.* I know better than to subject myself to that confusing hell hole. I'd heard too many horror stories of women being mistreated in dangerous and emotionally damaging ways at the ER during a miscarriage. It seems they only know what to do with women who show up with a *live* baby in their uterus. Even many medical professionals avoid facing the reality of pregnancy loss. Or, perhaps, it is their own discomfort with loss that leads them to shame patients as if the individual mother is to blame.

The previous weekend, when I was denied at urgent care for a RhoGAM shot, the urgency room also tried to block me completely, but I refused to leave without first speaking with a nurse. She made it clear that they would only give me the shot if I agreed to a complete exam. Another invasive ultrasound to "prove" that I was indeed having a miscarriage? Did they think I was lying? It was already in my chart that there was no heartbeat. Why couldn't the first one confirming there was no heartbeat, and the instructions from the doctor to seek out a RhoGAM, be enough? Without another word, I had turned and sprinted out the door, sobbing in my car, before the nurse could even finish her cold sentence.

This pregnancy loss is an overwhelming medical ordeal, a constant churn of advocating for myself and needing to be on top of every component. And I'm *good* at planning things, seeing the big picture, and managing details. I wasn't even new to this self-advocacy role, and it was still beyond exhausting. And expensive. A RhoGAM shot and other care were covered by insurance during pregnancy. I knew this from previous experience. But, if my baby was dead? I had to pay out of pocket. The bills showed up weeks to months later, delivering a new round of freshly cut grief. No ER!

My three- and five-year-old daughters are coming home soon. I need to be available for them. They need their mother.

Have I failed as a mother? Who am I as a mother if I can't keep a pregnancy? What does this mean for my two living daughters? What if I can't give them another sibling? Grief consumes me. Its familiar heaviness fills my chest and soon my entire body, sifting through my veins as if taking up permanent residence in every cell of my being. I feel a weight building. I've been able to shield my girls from this grief for the most part. But this time, it is simply too big. They are old enough now to know their mama is sick. I don't want this to be their grief too.

I won't go to the ER. I don't need it. Power through this, Katie. It's just like all those long-distance runs you've trained for. Yes, when I trained, there was a period when I always wanted to quit more than anything. *If I just keep going, I'll get to the finish line.*

My husband gets me a Gatorade and sits with me for a bit. I'm grateful. He would stay here the whole time and not leave my side if he could. He has consistently been a calm presence when I've needed it, and gives me space to sit with my pain. And we have the actual pressure of work to complicate the situation. We both have jobs to keep working, and we know our two girls will suffer if he stops. This is America. We work while we are miscarrying.

I close my eyes, breathing through the pain, and remind myself: *Don't hyperventilate, it will only make it worse. Stop shaking. Breathe.*

My mind, seeking something else to tether to, floats back to my first miscarriage.

Until it happened, I was blissfully unaware hell existed in this way. I mean, I'd heard first-hand accounts of others' miscarriages, and I'd had a healthy, successful first pregnancy with our daughter. She was a forty-one-weeker, and I chose to be induced. I planned my way through that. I was 100 percent sure of my dates, and when her due date came and went, I confidently accepted an induction offer from my doctor, showed up at the hospital that morning freshly showered, hair pulled back in a neat ponytail, all my planned-out hospital gear in tow, my long-distance running brain on, ready to cross the finish line with my beautiful, healthy baby in my arms. She arrived with speed in the end, but it otherwise went well. I had exercised my entire pregnancy. Heck, I had even lifted weights until thirty-six weeks! I was in the best shape of my life when I got pregnant with her—and continued to be after she was born.

I did what I was supposed to do.

Sure, the second pregnancy was a surprise. We were apprehensive of the timing, given our daughter was only fifteen months old. We hadn't planned for this. Nevertheless, we were excited.

I was still in good shape! I went for a run on Christmas Eve! Oh, wait . . . I had too much energy, didn't I? *Oh no.*

We had just arrived for Christmas dinner at my in-laws' house after spending the day with my family and our toddler. Shortly after arriving, I realized I was spotting. After what seemed like ages in the bathroom, my husband came looking for me. "We need to go outside. Now." We climbed into our car for privacy, cranking the engine to get some heat going and keep us from freezing in the Minnesota winter. I noticed the snow glittering on the car's hood as the Christmas moon shone. I made a phone call to the after-hours line, my hands shaking from the cold.

I told the triage nurse I needed the on-call OB-GYN to call me back.

I waited.

My phone eventually rang.

Voice cracking, I answered. "Hello? I'm about six weeks pregnant, and I am having spotting. I'm not sure what I should do," I explained with apprehension.

"You are probably having a miscarriage." The on-call doctor's short tone felt like a fiery slap on my cold face. "Go to the ER if the bleeding gets out of control."

Click.

I blinked in shock. *What?* She didn't even look at my chart. She doesn't know I'm Rh-negative and that I need a RhoGAM shot.

Maybe it's just some spotting, I reasoned with myself. *What am I supposed to do now?*

I turned to my husband. "I . . . I think we need to go home." He agreed, leaving the car's warmth to collect our daughter.

At home, under the twinkling lights of our Christmas tree, I snuggled our daughter and read her a book while wiping away my own tears. I focused on being the mother she needed in that moment and then hugged her tight, kissed her on the forehead, and stuffed down any remaining fear.

Yet, I couldn't ignore the growing cramps in my pelvis. I had no idea what was ahead. And was filled with utter dread.

What kind of Merry Christmas is this?

Overnight, I spent hours in the bathroom. As the pain wore on, I had a heartbreakingly stark realization: *I've known this before. My body knows this. This is far beyond period-like cramping. This is labor.*

Excruciating pain swelled deep in my pelvis, accompanied by bleeding and increasing nausea; as the pain grew, so did the bleeding. Consumed by a complete feeling of . . . loss, I doubled over from blood clots and uncontrollable nausea. I closed my eyes, attempting to do a calming yoga breath, but instead, I couldn't stop shaking uncontrollably and trying not to vomit. I hate vomiting. I spent the rest of the night alone in the bathroom in the dark, the only light coming from the glow of the Christmas moon through the window.

The following day, I called the clinic, knowing I needed to see my doctor as soon as possible, even though the on-call doctor gave no further instructions the prior evening. At the clinic, my doctor confirmed I was having a miscarriage. She was gracious and compassionate and ordered a RhoGAM without me having to ask. Every detail was handled, and she outlined what I needed to do next, including blood draws to track my hCG pregnancy hormone levels to zero. My doctor was *the* example of a calm, caring, experienced professional who knew how to handle a difficult situation with grace and dignity. And I was so grateful.

My mom had come to watch our daughter so my husband could accompany me. He could only join me because Christmas was a Sunday that year, and Monday was the holiday. Otherwise, he likely would have had to go to work because we didn't have time flexibility. We were "grateful" this occurred during his break from law school.

A jolt of pain pulls me back into the present on the bathroom floor, back into this fourth loss. *Breathe . . . through the pain.* I consider whether the immediate danger has passed. *Maybe I don't need to go to the ER?* If I can stay hydrated, the worst of it might be over. This has been building for a week and a half since I first found out this pregnancy wasn't viable. I closed my eyes and visualized the stages of a long-distance run. The build up—that first mile was always the biggest mental hurdle. After I crossed mile three, I could keep on sailing.

I think I'm past mile three now. I've got this. I'm confident I'm in the home stretch. No ER.

My husband picks up the kids from daycare. Despite my attempts to make it to the couch, increased bleeding quickly sends me back to the bathroom floor. I'm trapped by what is happening in my body.

My five-year-old—empathic and wise beyond her years—is skipping down the hall to greet me. Smiling, I want nothing more in this moment than to see my beautiful girls and their bright faces ready for hugs and kisses. Still, I stay lying on the floor, peering up at her, trying not to activate further nausea.

"It's OK, Mommy. You are going to be OK," she says, smiling at me with soft, sage confidence. I'm engulfed in a wave of gratitude for this tiny human, her large, caring spirit, her kind, inclusive heart. And at the same time, my heart is instantly heavy. She's from the before times. Before loss. Before trauma. Before . . . so much. My ray of sunshine. I am clinging to her energy. I'm becoming keenly aware that she now carries a piece of me that I fear no longer exists.

I'm beyond grateful to be her mom.

Mom. I have two daughters now. I'm so grateful I get to be a mother and that they are here with me—one from before and one from after . . . the first two miscarriages. We wanted to give them another sibling, but this is now two more losses in three months. I don't know if I can do this again. And yet, for them? I would do anything.

After all, becoming a mother transformed me in ways I could never have imagined. So has loss.

And this loss—this grief of recurrent pregnancy loss without explanation—is enormous. I feel it cumulating from the past three miscarriages. I'm not sure how I will contain it this time. I feel myself questioning how it is possible to approach something this big with my daughters. They are still so small. They need their mama. This stage of parenting is so . . . physical. And I'm so sick.

Will this ever end? I am desperately pondering this as I again sink into the familiar space on the tile. This whole thing is so lonely. Miscarriage is not *that* uncommon, I know this now, and yet on my fourth round of this, I still find it endlessly isolating and confusing to navigate. I'm a planner by nature, I self-advocate, and I am well-educated regarding fertility, pregnancy, and miscarriage. And it takes so much energy to manage this. I find it endlessly frustrating and ironic that there are standards for bringing life into the world, but with loss, it is lonely, exhausting, and grossly full of shame.

Closing my eyes, I breathe again. A slow, deep breath, filling my lungs to capacity, reaching my diaphragm. My breath is heavy with emotion. I hold it for a moment. As I slowly release, I attempt to bring calm to my shaking body, and I revisit how I got here.

My third miscarriage is still *so* fresh in my mind, having occurred only a few months prior. And yet, this fourth one is the worst by far in every way; physically, emotionally, and I seem to be lacking energy with every passing day. And what little energy I do have is consumed with an all too familiar feeling: grief. I know now to let it be—to carry it, because I know from experience it won't do me any good to bury it. Grief is not something we "get over." Yet, I feel its weight growing like a heavy chain—link by link—around my body. Each loss, each life experience altered, every future plan erased, the chain grows longer and heavier. Grief is now inextricably woven into my journey as a mother.

Four losses now. Four times I've kept life moving at home, at work, and within me, all while this grief chain continues to grow. Our plans for what we thought our life would be shifts by the day. How I show up in mom conversations at preschool drop off and pick up, at daycare, and beyond, now feels . . . guarded. Secondary losses—plans and social connections. And, yet, there is also joy. I reflect on how I've learned to weave pockets of joy into these devastating grief chasms that accompany each loss. I am now keenly aware of how much it matters. Despite my proactive attempts, I can't plan my way out of a miscarriage. And, I do get to choose how to respond. Joy doesn't erase the grief and pain, but it offers welcome glimmers of relief. I think about my first miscarriage and the first way I created a pocket of joy; miscarriage soup.

I could hardly eat. I was only days into the loss, and so ill and weak. I dragged myself to a work lunch I felt I "should" go to. And I made sure to choose the restaurant, my favorite bistro—a cozy spot run by an Austrian chef that was my neighborhood slice of Europe. I knew Chef had homemade chicken noodle soup on the menu, which I could fathom I had a decent chance of actually eating. It was the first meal I had finished in days. Every bit of warmth it delivered nourished me to my core. After that, I referred to it as "miscarriage soup." I will never again take for granted the power of some broth, chicken, and quality vegetables for the soul and the body.

It was a pocket of simple joy within the grief and heartache—a relief, a release, and a lesson learned that even though I desperately tried to figure out my way through this unexpected loss and a professional commitment, I could choose how to respond. Miscarriage soup. A simple joy.

Five years have passed between my first conscious simple joy and this fourth loss. I had miscarriage soup last week. My mom got it for me immediately following the devastating ultrasound news that this pregnancy wasn't viable. It didn't change anything about the outcome. And, I now choose how to respond. Now, I can plan how I respond, and I know how much feeling normal, and choosing a pocket of joy matters in what's to come.

I close my eyes and breathe through a new round of pain deep in my pelvis, reflecting on the lessons I've learned.

My second miscarriage. Only a few months after my first one. Where I learned about choosing gratitude in the depths of loss. Not grateful that I was experiencing it, but that it was over fast and that I was spared miscarriage illness, unlike my first one, which rendered me sick for weeks.

I chuckle to myself, remembering that I wasn't spared all illness though. It is a fresh layer of hell being in a two-week wait to take a pregnancy test while facing a stomach bug that our toddler brought home from daycare. That pregnancy was over as quickly as the stomach bug extricated itself from my system. I call it grief gratitude. It doesn't erase an ounce of grief. Yet, I can choose to add in bits of solace. Pockets of normalcy. Simple joy.

And I did just that with my second miscarriage. I so badly wanted life to continue normally, and so I still hosted our friends to watch our high school play in the state hockey tournament that weekend. This is Minnesota where high school hockey rivals college teams in many places.

Friends and hockey. Another pocket of joy.

And yet, none of our guests knew what I had been through that week. That was the first time I remember feeling lonely around longtime friends. My whole world had changed. It was no longer an isolated miscarriage. This second one, rapidly as it occurred, meant I needed to see my doctor.

Who was I kidding? Normal, as I knew it, was already gone. I just couldn't admit it yet.

This invisible, massively isolating grief was stacking like a brick wall. A wall I was subconsciously building to keep myself safe.

While our friends drank beer, ate snacks, gathered in our cozy living room, and cheered on our high school, I began mulling over raw data in my head and activating a plan. I knew, based on all the cycle charting I'd been doing—alarm going off at 5:45 every morning, rolling over, taking my temperature with a basal body thermometer, and later logging that data in my fertility chart—that it was time to address further fertility interventions. I'd been charting my cycles for years now. I had solid data showing that the luteal phase—the second half—of my cycle often ran too short to sustain a pregnancy.

I open my eyes again, back in the midst of my current pain. The early spring sun softly glows through the window. The mirror lights are exceedingly bright. *Gosh, this floor is hard. And cold.* Even a blanket isn't helping. My back hurts.

I don't know if I can do this again. I worked so hard to have our second daughter after that second loss. Every single detail was managed, planned, and executed. There was no ease in it. I had started acupuncture along with the cooperation of my doctor in an effort to avoid taking fertility meds. My acupuncturist gave me a list of things we would do to ensure a solid, strong ovulation, including knocking back royal jelly. It was gross. And worth it. I diligently took it until I ovulated. I did acupuncture the entire pregnancy. I got on progesterone as soon as I had a positive test. The glaring reality is that I would not have my beautiful rainbow baby without my acupuncturist. I'm forever grateful.

I planned my way through the whole thing—and it worked. It also cost me a lot. A few months into that pregnancy, I was emotionally crumbling. Extreme stress oozed out of me everywhere. Work stress, at-home stress, pregnancy stress. Pressure from colleagues, family, and friends to "be more open" even when we asked for privacy. Which was even more isolating.

Was I going to deliver a live or dead baby?

The question plagued me constantly. I had lost all trust that my body would see this through. Even with the pockets of joy I consciously created with our toddler, managing it became overwhelming. As the days passed and my belly grew, pressure from outside opinions mounted. It was increasingly hard to maintain the privacy I so desperately sought. After all, I was still a person, not a delivery mechanism for any baby—dead or alive. I could still be me, and also be growing this human. *Why was this concept so hard to grasp?* Why did all these people have an opinion on how I should act during this stressful and personal time? And why did they feel it is *ever* okay to comment on the state of a woman's uterus? I could not ignore the irony of our culture's "hush-hush" approach to miscarriage, as if the woman is to blame, and the deep offense one causes in imploring privacy during a full-term pregnancy. Thankfully, my husband and immediate family's calm support kept me afloat.

And it wasn't enough. Fear and stress were consuming me. Three months into the pregnancy, my doctor referred me to a therapist. She knew me well enough at this point to know I do not take life passively—I proactively lead my own life, I *will* self-advocate, and I was drowning with the extreme stress load I was carrying. It was time to learn that even with all the proactive planning skills, it *is* okay to ask for help. This therapist was the right person at the right time. I could not see how desperately I needed a safe space to guide me through the remainder of that pregnancy. And to navigate all the opinions and demands coming at me from so many directions. Her guidance became a true pocket of joy, as she also taught me one of the biggest self-advocacy lessons of all; the value of taking a break. I had attempted to plan my way through everything, and it would do me no good if I reached the finish line completely burned out.

At thirty-eight weeks pregnant, I had landed in the hospital with concerns about decreased fetal movement after leading a big work event, and managing a lot of unnecessary chaos behind the scenes. This therapist insisted I stop working for the remainder of the pregnancy. *After all, I still wouldn't let myself believe I was going to deliver a live baby.* Fear was blocking joy and hope. I was in no shape to give birth, as I was still not convinced my body was going to complete this immense task, even with the previous smooth delivery of our oldest daughter. Grief, stress, and self-distraction were consuming me. I seriously needed to get out of my own way, and she guided me there. That brief period I stepped back from work before having my second daughter was a gift of time I could *never* have pulled together on my own, even with being a big-picture and details-oriented planner. I'm forever grateful for her guidance and insistence, and I learned a valuable lesson that I often share with other women facing stressful life events: seeking help is not weak. It is strong. It is wise. And so many women further down the path in life are willing to extend a hand to others, if you let them, as if saying, "I've got you. I've been there too. You are not alone. Keep going."

While being deeply immersed in this fourth loss, I feel growing gratitude for the women before me who shared their stories of pain, loss, and recovery. I couldn't fully articulate it; that would come with time and healing wisdom. But I was becoming more conscious of choosing gratitude in these harrowing moments the way I already had—with things like miscarriage soup. While embracing the immense physical and emotional pain, I was unlearning that emotions might be mutually exclusive. It *is* possible to be engulfed in simultaneous deep pain *and* deep joy. I realized consciously that I feel this every day with my daughters. The duality of the emotions floods me. I could be despondent about what I was facing. And so grateful for the extra quiet time with my daughters. When the nausea would finally subside a bit, I could join them on the couch for snuggles and watch Doc McStuffins. I could be terrified of facing what was ahead in trying to recover from this miscarriage. And immensely calm about knowing I would find a way. I had done this before. I was beginning to lean into the wisdom of experience. And with the deep knowledge and expertise I now carry, knowing we won't ever go back to before. I'll never again have that innocence of a first pregnancy without fear. And that is okay to grieve. Life does move forward, not on. Forward.

I am gutted physically, mentally, and emotionally—and yet, the awareness and gratitude for the women who have survived this before me and who shared their stories moves me. I am not alone. As I gaze at the white marble tile on the bathroom wall I personally remodeled, I think about friends who have shared their own miscarriage stories with me, as well as acquaintances I have met online who are also walking the same painful path. I silently thank my doctor, who has guided me more than once, through what was to come and treated me with postpartum respect in the aftermath. My heart fills with gratitude for my therapist for gently teaching me about grief and holding space for the losses I had experienced. Even if it was an invisible loss to many, it wasn't to her. My acupuncturist, who would diligently begin restoring strength to my body as soon as I could visit her. The weight of this gratitude swells with every passing minute, and for the first time, I consciously feel less alone, realizing how much we need to lean into our intuition as women and mothers to speak up and self-advocate *and* also to extend a hand to others.

I lean into the memory of my grandmother, who raised her children in this very house where I lay on the bathroom floor, and whose presence I feel regularly through revisiting her lessons and stories. Most importantly to me, how she shared the story of her three-month-old baby who died due to a heart condition in the 1950s; something that, today, could be fixed. She knew something was wrong, being her third baby, but was repeatedly dismissed by doctors. Her mother's intuition was deep. The way I know deep in my soul that the signs were there from the beginning—this last pregnancy was not viable. In choosing to share this story with me, she planted seeds I would use many years later to advocate for myself through each loss. I breathe her spirit in, channeling her wisdom, as my understanding of the pain she carried deepens by the moment.

As I continue riding out this last loss, eventually, the nausea breaks enough, and I'm able to curl up with a blanket on the couch and snuggle with my daughters. I close my eyes, revisiting this emotional journey. From the pure joy of my two daughters to the deep valleys of four losses. After a series of confusing medical events over the past two years: shingles, my back going out, ovulation pain so intense I told my doctor I wanted to rip out my ovaries, increasing fatigue, all with no explanation and a clean bill of health, slapped dismissively at me by an endocrinologist, I had convinced myself that my cycles were okay enough not to warrant so many carefully planned interventions.

Following the arrival of our rainbow baby, our rainbow after the storm, we *so* wanted to have a third child. And I tried to relax my plan-every-detail approach. After all, managing two kids, a full-time job, and growing medical confusion was a lot. And now I have miscarriages three and four to go with it and a whole lot more confusion.

I take a slow, deep breath, channeling my own wisdom now. I know I have a more prolonged recovery ahead than I want to admit. I have experienced this three times previously and this time is . . . intense.

Later, that intensity turned out to be a sign. My body had been screaming at me that something was wrong. And I realized, in that time on the bathroom floor, things started to shift in me; physically and emotionally. Initially, it was relief. As I snuggled on the couch with my daughters, I soaked up every bit of joy from slowing down to be with my girls while recovering. But relief turned into reflection. I had now become vastly more educated on listening to my body, and I was conscious of this. And though I was hopeful it was time to heal, the spring events would soon explain much of my other confusing medical symptoms. The increasing nausea, pain, fatigue, and other signs of malaise were actually cancer—an extremely rare, well-differentiated papillary mesothelioma of the peritoneum. It was found in the abdominal cavity behind my uterus during an exploratory surgery later that summer, seeking an explanation for the growing symptoms that had plagued me even more intensely that spring, following that last loss. Physically, my body had been telling me there was more. And I had to channel my inner wisdom, with the guidance of the support team of women I had unknowingly been building—my therapist, doctor, and acupuncturist—to advocate for further action.

Emotionally, I was shifting into a knowing that this was the end of my fertility journey. I couldn't yet articulate it, but I was learning to listen to my inner wisdom as a woman and a mother. There was no neat conclusion to this, wrapped up in a bow. I didn't get to bring home a third sibling for my daughters. I didn't even lose the option. Life took a drastic shift, and it just ended.

Every day, I am reminded that I can choose how to respond to this heartache. This changed my identity as a mother. I might not have been here, and I might not have had the chance to be a mother. I get to choose every day how to respond to what life tosses our way, and what path to forge next.

I've been pregnant six times. I have two living daughters. I'm cancer-free and grateful to be alive. I'm thankful to get to raise my girls. For the beautiful memories and for being here to help them navigate the hard times. And while I carry each pregnancy in my heart always, and the grief alongside, I also live with daily reminders of this heartache—of the loss I carry in my heart and how this affects our family.

I deeply grasp what it's like to be a mother before loss, what it's like to have a successful pregnancy after loss, and the stark reality of a fertility journey abruptly halting without resolution.

And, it also turns out that when the path you thought you were on in life goes up in flames, it can result in true freedom. I'm not bound by the shoulds as a mother. I broke up with trying to plan my way through everything. I make space for true, deep joy, amid real, lasting emotional pain.

Sometimes this means going on another Walt Disney World vacation, because of the joy, escape, and fabulous memories we've made. It includes leaning into mom conversations where I can hold space for another woman going through her own tragedy, and politely passing on other social gatherings focused on mom conversations that take the ability to be a mom for granted. Other times, it means declining activities tailored to larger families with younger children in pursuit of experiences like live community theatre and multi-age programs such as our Irish dance school. Activities that allow space for us to live alongside our grief and escape to our cabin in northern Minnesota to soak up a different pace of life. These are all decisions—including purchasing that cabin—that would have had a different outcome without loss.

That doesn't negate the grief and the pain. It just . . . is.

Every single thing I do as a mother—all the memories we've made because of things we could do as a family of four instead of five, and all the things we will miss out on not being a family of five—is layered with grief. Every day I get the choice to lean into yes, and. Not yes, but.

Sometimes, I fail.

And then I remember that yes, and . . . deep pain and deep joy do coexist.

Bio

Katie Jamieson is a multifaceted travel entrepreneur, speaker, author, and association/nonprofit leader dedicated to connecting, inspiring, and uplifting others. As the CEO and founder of Engage! Travel Co., a full-service travel agency, and Engage! Community Building for Nonprofits in St. Paul, Minnesota, Katie brings her visionary approach, detail-oriented action, and unwavering commitment to every project she leads. Her philosophy of putting good back into the world shines through in her leadership style, client engagement, and how she grows and engages her team. Passionate about integrating travel and life, Katie has traveled extensively domestically and abroad, leveraging this experience, and her signature phrase, travel with life, into every vacation her team serves.

With decades of experience leading nonprofit programs and associations, leading professional continuing education certification programs, inspiring the next generation of STEM professionals, and navigating organizational change as an executive director, Katie excels at empowering organizations to thrive. Her personal experiences with self-advocacy, loss, overcoming life-altering medical challenges, and navigating deep joys and pains enrich her keynotes and writings, making them resonate deeply with audiences. Whether she's planning memorable vacations or consulting for nonprofits, Katie's work is infused with a commitment to lead and serve with gratitude. Learn more about working with Katie or inquire about speaking engagements at www.katiejamieson.com.

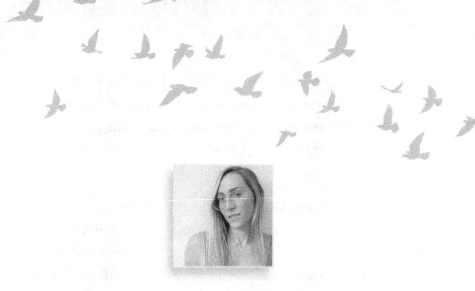

SOUL CONTRACT

Carrie Averett

I'll never forget one of the most important conversations of my life. I was in my early twenties and home for the summer. Or was it late spring and I was getting treatment at the hospital? Those years are such a blur in my memory as I navigated health issue after health issue. Either way, I was spending the evening with my chosen family—my boyfriend, his sister, and their loving father Bill.

Bill had always been a father figure to me, even before my father passed. He was everything my father wasn't—kind, loving, full of insight, and emotionally present in a way most men I've met struggle to be.

"Want to go for a walk?" Bill asked us after dinner. Taking late-night walks to the graveyard in their neighborhood became a type of ritual for all of us over the years. We'd each grab a drink and go stargazing while we chatted about life. "I'm too tired tonight," both my boyfriend and his sister said in unison, letting out rather obnoxious yawns.

"I'll go," I responded, softly smiling back at Bill. Admittingly, I loved the times he and I got to connect one-on-one. He was one of the few people who really saw me at a time in my life when I craved to be seen. Our relationship was one I never had with my own father, and I cherished it greatly.

I can still feel the warm Baltimore breeze that night as we made our way to the graveyard. We both sat down and looked up at the dark sky. I think the graveyard is still, in my mind, one of my favorite places—somewhere I could always retreat to when my world got too loud, which was often.

"How are you doing?" Bill asked me as his eyes scanned the stars above us.

"I'm okay, I guess," I responded. He waited for me to elaborate. "I just feel a little lost right now, I think," I began. "It feels like everyone else I know is doing what they're 'supposed' to do, you know? Graduate high school, go to college, study hard and party harder, graduate college, get an adult job and make lots of money, marry your partner, adopt a dog, eventually have a baby or two, join a country club, and live happily ever after," I finished off the list with a fake smile that suggested my feelings all too well.

"And how does that trajectory make you feel, Carrie?" he quipped back.

"Honestly?" I responded. "It makes me want to run as fast and as far away as humanly possible." He let out a giant laugh that seemed to both surprise and delight him. I laughed too. "It just seems like everyone is checking all of these boxes, you know? And I . . . I just don't want to live that way. . . . I don't think I could live that way if I tried," I trailed on.

Bill sat quiet for a moment, taking in my words.

"You know, time and age are not linear," he eventually said.

I sat silently, waiting for him to explain.

"You don't have to follow the same timeline as your friends if it doesn't feel like it's right for you. You can do things your own way in your own order if you want."

I sat with that statement for a minute and decided it was more than just words. It was permission for me to take the biggest exhale.

It started when I was twelve; I realized I was different from those around me. Mainly because I spent years in and out of hospitals with doctors trying to figure out why my stomach hurt all the time. It hurt to eat, hurt to move, hurt to play with my friends the way most middle schoolers did with ease. As a result, I constantly felt anxious. *What was wrong with me? And why couldn't the adults figure it out?*

I was eventually diagnosed with Crohn's disease and then polycystic ovary syndrome (PCOS), which offered some comfort—simply having an explanation for my exhaustion and pain was validating—but those years changed me irrevocably. Not only did my grit strengthen, but I also developed a curiosity around death and spirituality, which seemed fitting for a kid who was undergoing major surgeries.

I remember having a conversation with my eighth grade religion teacher after class one day. "I keep getting hospitalized and need to know: is it safe to die?" I asked her.

She looked back at me with the type of gentle expression only the safest of teachers can give. "Here's what I can tell you, sweetie. You're absolutely going to be okay. Whenever your soul feels like it's time for you to go—*whenever* that is—you will be protected."

While I recognize now that some adults may have found her response to be inappropriate, I was and still am deeply grateful for it. She helped me realize I didn't have to be afraid, that I could find peace in the unknown.

I felt that peace again in my conversation with Bill all these years later. *I don't have to follow the same timeline as those around me. Whatever I chose, I would be okay.*

That night Bill offered me a permission slip to pave my own path, an opened door to liberation. *Time and age are not linear.* His words resounded in my mind the rest of the night. It would take years for me to fully grasp their meaning.

I remember everything about the day I found out I was pregnant. I was in my late twenties, at work wearing some insane yoga outfit, and I felt this new, unusual sensation in my body. I waited for my lunch break and bolted for the nearest CVS to get a pregnancy test.

Oh God, I hope no one I know sees me buying this, I thought to myself as I pulled the box from the shelf as discreetly as I could. I paid for the tests, and ran back to work faster than a bat out of hell. I flung the bathroom door open, and frantically read the directions. I peed on the stick, started the countdown, and paced back and forth across the large single bathroom. *Fifteen minutes.* That was all that was left between the *now* of my life and whatever the *future* was going to bring.

How could this be happening? I agonized as I paced. Because I had been diagnosed with PCOS when I was a young teenager, I hadn't had a consistent period in years. As the timer ticked down to nine minutes, all I could think about was how my partner would respond. *What would he say? Would this ruin our plans?*

Wait, is that one line or two? I picked up the stick to get a closer look. It appeared to be two little lines in pink in the tiny window on the stick. *I need a second opinion to be sure.* I sent a photo to my best friend for confirmation. The kit had two tests, so she encouraged me to take the other one. I had heard of false positives, and I was desperately praying that was the case.

I can't be pregnant right now.

I can't be pregnant right now.

I can't be pregnant right now.

Two more pink lines. *Fuck.*

I was definitely pregnant.

My now ex, life partner at the time, did not want to have children and honestly, I was okay with that. I was young, and he was this cool, alternative guy that worked in the music industry. Between tour life and his challenging relationship with his own father, I understood that being a dad wasn't exactly high on his bucket list.

We had discussed it, and both decided we were going to live a full, adventurous lifestyle together instead, a path of our very own creation. One where we didn't live to work, but rather worked to live. Our priority wasn't to make more money like so many others, but rather to experience life to the fullest. That meant traveling freely, hiking and camping through national parks, and just being present and available to all that was here in the now.

I was willing to understand that choosing this alternative life probably meant missing out on other experiences like motherhood, at least in the traditional sense. And at the time, I thought I was good with that.

I held on to the belief that all I was gaining in my relationship would make up for what I was losing.

I will never forget the amount of love I received that night while I cried in his arms, telling him that we were pregnant. I was terrified to have that conversation because I didn't want to ruin anything between us. He looked into my swollen eyes and said, "The next time that this happens, my love, it will be on purpose, and we will celebrate." I cried even more as I looked deeply at him. His words comforted me. *Perhaps the door wasn't completely closed to us having children in the future. Time and age are not linear.*

And then I realized what he had not said but I knew anyway—I would be getting an abortion.

Looking back, I can't believe we didn't really talk about it. The decision was made more or less through a shared look—a brief exchange of silent understanding. We were young and feared that bringing a child into the picture before we were ready would have ruined our lives. He was my person and we believed we would be bonded forever, and so I gave up what could have been our child for the sake of our relationship, for the sake of our future.

We didn't know it then, but this would be the only chance for me to physically carry a child in this lifetime, a grief that still visits me frequently.

About a year later, I started to get sick. *Really sick.* Months went by and once again doctors were unable to figure out what was going on. Countless late nights turned into even longer days spent at the ER, and they always ended in the same way: there was nothing wrong with me. It was medical gaslighting at its finest, and I was growing impatient.

My cells were mutating, and my body was noticeably beginning to change. I remember one evening being startled when I looked down at my legs—they were full of fluid which I eventually learned was lymphedema. I was forced to wobble through the snow in flip-flops because they were the only shoes that would fit my swollen feet, to the only place I would go those days: back to the ER. Through gritted teeth, I demanded that they drain the fluid from my feet and test it. I was in such excruciating pain that I threatened to puncture it myself if they wouldn't do it. I watched the nurses share aggravated glances at each other, but I was too angry to care. Finally, they admitted me. I was desperate and the only way I could think to get their attention was to threaten my own self-harm. *What a system.*

After months of unbearable pain and endless questions, I finally got my answer.

"Are you Carrie?" a doctor asked me as I made my way out of the hospital one late evening, feeling completely depleted. I nodded my head yes, and he kindly introduced himself to me as my hematologist. "I believe I know what is wrong with you. I want to schedule a bone marrow biopsy first thing tomorrow morning." I agreed to the test, willing to try anything, and thanked him for helping. Over the next few days my life changed irrevocably.

After the bone marrow biopsy, I received a phone call. "Hey Carrie, I'm calling to let you know we have your test results, you have a blood cancer called acute myeloid leukemia. AML for short." Time stood still. I was in complete shock. I had just celebrated my twenty-ninth birthday. *How could this be happening? How could I be getting sick again?*

My partner and I sat on the stairs of our Baltimore city home and were silent for what felt like a lifetime after I got off the call. *My cancer diagnosis.* Definitely *not* a part of the plan.

And then just like that, time sped up, and things moved extremely fast. We went into survival mode and carefully created my support team.

"I'll take off work as much as I can and take care of you," my partner promised, optimistic in his abilities to show up selflessly for me, *for us.* It would become the ultimate death sentence for our relationship. "And when I'm on tour," he continued, "our friends and family will step in to help." Our home, once a safe haven for peace and dreaming up our future plans, quickly morphed into a space of chaos and dis-ease.[1] I began undergoing aggressive treatments of chemotherapy immediately, and endured full body radiation that just about fried every ounce of my insides, including my brain.

I'd make my way into our bathroom many nights, look in the mirror, and think: *Who is she?*

I felt like that little twelve-year-old girl all over again; it hurt to eat, hurt to move, hurt to play the way my friends played so effortlessly. And yet, my body also felt like it had aged fifty years overnight. To make matters more challenging, I was also placed into medically induced menopause. I felt simultaneously young and extremely old, like I was living on multiple timelines. And worst of all, I felt so alone. And even though we never talked about it, I know my partner did too. Our lives had become so isolated in efforts to keep me safe from everyday sicknesses that my body couldn't easily ward off. Our world, once big and full of possibility, now seemed so small.

---

1   A state of unease and imbalance between one's body, mind, and spirit.

My partner tried to take my mind off the hardships of the present by projecting into the future. We'd talk about us getting married sooner rather than later, what our wedding would look like, how we'd travel to new countries, and all the adventures we would have together. He and I both held tightly to that vision. Most of the time it was the only thing that got us through the dark days. It was our survival guide.

After many treatments of chemotherapy, my team of doctors and I realized we were not getting our desired result. The greatest chance I had for recovery, they explained, was a full bone marrow transplant. It was at this time that I learned just how challenging it would be for me to ever have children, a conversation that without question should have happened before I started cancer treatment, yet didn't; it was another unspoken conversation that would forever impact my life. There my partner and I were, learning about IVF right before I was scheduled to get a bone marrow transplant to save my life. If we wanted any chance of having our own child one day, this was our only option. My body had already undergone so much. *How hard could IVF be?*

My partner and I walked into the office of our infertility doctor, and began the learning process. We were quickly told the pros and cons of freezing eggs and creating embryos. We had planned to get married so this felt like an easy decision. I still remember our doctor asking, and us looking into each other's eyes, smiling, and saying at the same time: "embryos." My heart felt full knowing that we had a backup plan should we ever want children of our own one day. It's funny, we rarely ever talked about children before this, but I was grateful that he agreed to keep the door open in case I ever wanted us to have that kind of family.

In the end we were able to create one single embryo. *That's it?*

That's it.

At the same time, so many of our loved ones were actually getting married and starting families. I remember waking up groggy in the middle of the day posttreatment and looking over at my phone to read messages announcing, "I have news—we're engaged!" and "Guess what? I'm pregnant!"

I desperately wanted to be happy for my people and the lives they were creating for themselves, and I was; but when you are hanging on by a thread and have only one single embryo as your only option at possibly bearing your own child, it's hard not to feel painfully envious. I know my friends and family had compassion for me as I battled leukemia, but I don't think they fully realized the grief I was also experiencing. The truth is—the hardest part of cancer are the years following it and coming to terms with all that you have lost. I, myself, did not recognize how important motherhood was to me until I had the option taken away entirely. All I had wanted was an alternative way of living with my partner, but now it felt like my whole world was crumbling before me.

My life continued to unravel over the next two years. My partner grew more and more distant, spending time in different rooms than me and barely communicating; we no longer connected through our love and I began to brace myself for the worst.

"Carrie, I feel like we've been married for thirty years," he said to me one night as we sat on the couch watching a hockey game. The tension between us at that point was palpable. I could see the exhaustion on his face, dark circles had now weighed heavy under his eyes over the last year. "I just don't know if I can do this anymore. . . . I don't know if I want to," he confessed. He had stopped working, stopped spending time with his friends, and stopped enjoying life. Resentment now lived in his heart where there was once love. I could tell he didn't want to be the bad guy who broke up with his partner during cancer, but he was also losing himself. Feeling depleted from cancer, new emerging medical conditions from my transplant, and terrified of being abandoned in my darkest hour, I froze in that moment—motionless and without words.

He woke early the next morning and packed his suitcase. I didn't move when I heard the front door click open and then pull shut for a final time.

I spent years navigating a deep depression in the wake of his absence. I'd lie in my bed, covered with used tissues and old medication bottles, curtains drawn to block out the world, and try to make sense of the last few years of my life.

Pregnancy loss.
Cancer.
Chemo.
Isolation.
Radiation.
IVF.
Grief.
Bone marrow transplant.
Infertility.
Heartbreak.
Abandonment.
More grief.
The pandemic.
More isolation.
Loneliness.

It was a dark night of the soul paired with a total death of my life as I knew it.

Interestingly enough, when you get a full bone marrow transplant, your DNA is no longer traceable as your former self. While this might be sad for some, it was intoxicatingly freeing for me. For starters, on my cancerversary, to read *user not found* meant I was cancer-free. It's a rather unique experience and at the same time, it's the only thing that could ever make sense for my soul to exist not only in this body but beyond it. After years of knowing my life wouldn't look like the lives of those around me, of always feeling divinely pushed to pave my own path in a different direction, I felt validated. *This was my soul contract.* I was reminded of that conversation in the graveyard with Bill all those years ago. Here in front of me was a death, but also a rebirth—*an opened door to liberation.* And I had no choice but to walk through it.

And it was the hardest thing I've ever done. Harder than child loss, harder than cancer, harder than grief. To endure those losses and keep moving forward was the real work. First, I had to heal the dis-ease in my mind and soul that resulted from my cancer and all that came with it, including my infertility and heartbreak. I returned to my yoga mat, after fearing I wouldn't be able to, and I threw myself back into the practice. I started studying integrative yoga therapy which allowed me to work with my nervous system using tools such as breathwork, somatics, Mindfulness-Based Stress Reduction (MBSR), and meditation. I also embarked on what I called a *reclaiming year* for myself. I traveled once a month—usually somewhere new—and attended a concert once a week, inviting music to revitalize my spirit. I took up space intentionally and unapologetically. I spent time with people who made me happy and eventually I felt my pulse again.

I untethered myself from my old story—my outdated ego—and began to fall in love with my new life . . . just to be a soul truly floating free on this earth.

I felt the chaotic dust that surrounded me for so long begin to settle and noticed there was fertile soil underneath me. I felt truly grounded, situated in my own self, for the first time. I remembered that the only way to move forward is from this place.

After years of prioritizing my full recovery, I decided to reach out to my ex in hopes of finally discussing our past, and more importantly, the legal questions regarding our shared embryo. At first, he was extremely open to connecting and even dream-lining what our future co-parenting relationship could look like should I choose to have a surrogate carry our embryo.

I couldn't believe it. *Was this my silver lining?*

As hopeful as I was, I told him to pause and partner with his now-wife first, and he agreed that was the best next step. I hung up the phone and cried, feeling grateful that maybe I would get to experience motherhood afterall. Differently than I had initially imagined, but still—*motherhood.*

I called him a month later to check-in and he answered the phone with a stark, monotone voice that surprised me. That same darkness that swallowed me the morning he left all those years ago inched toward me once more.

"I feel so bad, Carrie," he began. "I have already taken so much from you in this lifetime." My heart stopped as I thought back to the wedding we dreamed about, and the travels, and all the plans we had made together. "I should have been more mindful when we first spoke, but I do not want any tether to that embryo. That's not my child." I almost dropped the phone, fearing I was going to be sick. *No, no, no, no, no, no. Why are you doing this?* I wanted to scream at him. Instead, I breathed through the rest of the conversation while fighting back tears. I feared that dark night of the soul was returning. I canceled my yoga classes, didn't go into work, and spent the day in the dark. I needed to numb myself in isolation in order to process. A voice inside me kept repeating *I can't go backward. I can't go back to having long days in the dark, curtains drawn, retreating from the world. Why would he want to intentionally cause me harm?*

The questions raced in circles around my head.

After taking a few days to process that heart-wrenching conversation alone, I turned to my support system of loved ones to help me through. I wish I could say that after some time, my ex and I came to an agreement regarding the rights to our shared embryo, but we're still navigating that whole legal process. As I write these words, I'm in this limbo of waiting to see what will happen next. It is not lost on me that we are living in an era where the conversation about women's agency over their bodies is so alive, and that story becomes even more complicated when you have a diagnosis of cancer and infertility, and shared rights to an embryo. In a way, it feels like my birthright as a woman to have my own child has been taken away many times over, which is why this grief is so heavy.

My own silver lining is that I have created alternative ways to mother in this lifetime. Being a mother doesn't have to mean giving birth to something with a physical heartbeat. I birthed my private practice The Flow, which specializes in integrative oncology and yoga therapy. I lead workshops and teacher trainings at local well-being studios, and also enjoy teaching an array of public yoga, somatics, breathwork, and meditation classes in my community. Through this work, I get to lovingly care for each and every one of my clients and patients, and help them remember their wholeness no matter what challenges they're navigating.

Because of my own lived experiences with the health care system, I have also devoted much of my life's work to helping bridge the gap between eastern and western medicine, emphasizing the importance of them both working together in partnership versus separately in order to take a whole-person approach to healthcare. I am grateful to now help pave the way for integrative oncology in clinical settings as a grant-funded yoga therapist at Baltimore's largest public hospital. I get to mother this emerging field and practice that will one day be covered by insurance nationwide.

Through working one-on-one with many oncology patients and their caregivers, I have often thought of my ex and the sacrifices he made in order to help keep me alive. It was challenging for me to have empathy for him while we were in the thick of our relationship ending, but now I can see how much suffering he endured as my caregiver. Having to give up so much of his life and the "normal" relationship he had initially signed on for must have been hard for him, his own grief to process. In one of our last conversations as a couple, he told me that everything he loved about me, about us, had become darkened with cancer. What a heartbreaking truth for us both.

And yet, it all led me here. *Cancer, menopause, infertility, IVF, isolation, heartbreak, abandonment.* It guided me to my soul contract, to my life's work, to my dharma as we say in the yoga world. To offer to others the comfort and support I so desperately craved on my darkest days; to be willing to have the challenging conversations with them, no matter how uncomfortable. To be seen not only as a cancer patient, but as a human being wanting to feel whole again. I think back to that moment with my eighth grade religion teacher, and it wasn't so much what she said, but how she made me feel that stayed with me. In a time of sickness and inner turmoil, she helped me find peace in the unknown, reminding me that no matter what, I would be okay.

And I was. And I am. And my story isn't over just yet. And so it is.

Carrie is a certified integrative yoga therapist and a thought leader among integrative oncology who is paving the way in hospitals for pediatric, adolescence, and young adult integrative healthcare. Inspired by her personal health journey to serve others, she is a mother to her own private yoga therapy practice, The Flow, in which she guides clients back into a state of balance and wholeness through using a holistic lens while navigating a medical diagnosis. Carrie helps support her local studios where she also offers public yoga therapeutic classes, somatics, breath work, meditation, Ayurveda, nidra, and more. She has over a thousand hours of additional training and certifications within the Eastern health & wellness realm. She loves to share her knowledge by leading workshops and teacher trainings.

Carrie is a community connector and is committed to helping support local women-owned businesses and nonprofits. Carrie has a mindfulness grant-funded job at Baltimore's largest public hospital, Sinai Hospital, as a yoga therapist where she works with pediatrics, adolescents and young adults, family members, and caregivers to help navigate all pathways of cancer. She is committed to continuing her education to help guide others one day as a certified Ayurvedic health counselor and end-of-life doula. Carrie sits on an oncology patient and faculty board at The Johns Hopkins Hospital and advocates for adolescent and young adult (AYA) cancer patients, helping to pave the way for integrative oncology.

With a diagnosis of leukemia at the age of twenty-nine, Carrie was thrust into not just a clinical diagnosis but a series of experiences that cracked her multidimensional being. She found and reclaimed her wholeness and is committed to helping others remember their wholeness too.

In an era where the conversation about women's agency over their bodies is so alive, the story becomes even more complicated when you have a diagnosis of cancer and infertility. A story and a conversation Carrie feels called to bring to light in service of others. *The Losses We Keep* is Carrie's first book. You can connect with Carrie and learn more about her work on Instagram @csavirett and reach her at info@theflowbaltimore.com and theflowbaltimore.com.

GLOSSARY OF KEY MEDICAL TERMS

Acute myeloid leukemia (AML). A fast-developing type of blood cancer that starts in the bone marrow—the soft inner part of bones where new blood cells grow.

Arthrogryposis. A condition present at birth where one or more of the joints are stuck in a fixed position, either straight or bent, and have limited movement; a group of disorders where multiple joints become stiff and immobile due to tight muscles and tendons that cause the joints to lock in place.

Bicornuate uterus. A condition present at birth where the uterus has a heart-shaped appearance instead of the typical pear shape. In this type of uterine malformation, the uterus has two joined cavities, while a normal uterus has just one.

Bone marrow transplant. A medical procedure where a doctor replaces damaged or diseased bone marrow with healthy bone marrow.

Cesarean section (C-section). A surgical procedure where an incision in the abdomen and uterus is used to deliver a baby. This is often done when a vaginal delivery isn't possible or safe for the mother or baby.

Crohn's disease. A chronic type of inflammatory bowel disease (IBD) that can affect any part of the gastrointestinal tract, but it most commonly impacts the end of the small intestine.

Dilation and curettage (D&C). A medical procedure where the cervix is widened and a tool is used to remove tissue from inside the uterus.

Down Syndrome. A genetic condition that is characterized by developmental delays and usually cognitive challenges ranging from minor to more significant. This condition is caused by having an extra copy of chromosome 21.

Ectopic pregnancy. When a fertilized egg develops outside the uterus, like in a fallopian tube or the abdominal cavity.

Endometrial Receptivity Analysis (ERA). A diagnostic test that helps determine the best time to transfer an embryo into a woman's uterus for implantation during an in vitro fertilization (IVF) cycle.

Euploid embryo. An embryo that has the correct number of chromosomes; this means the embryo has a chromosome number that is an exact multiple of the basic set of chromosomes, reducing the risk of genetic abnormalities.

External cephalic version (ECV or version). A medical procedure performed by a healthcare provider to reposition a fetus that is in a breech (bottom first or feet first) presentation. During an ECV, the doctor manually rotates the fetus into a headfirst (cephalic) position to facilitate a safer vaginal delivery. This procedure can help mitigate complications associated with breech births.

Gestational carrier (surrogate). A woman who becomes pregnant through artificial insemination or the implantation of an embryo created via in vitro fertilization (IVF), with the intention of carrying the pregnancy to term on behalf of another individual or couple.

Granulosa cell tumor (GCT). A type of ovarian tumor that originates from the granulosa cells, which are involved in the production of estrogen in the ovaries.

Hematologist. A doctor who specializes in blood conditions.

Hemoglobin. A protein in red blood cells that contains iron. It carries oxygen from the lungs to the rest of the body and helps return carbon dioxide from the body to the lungs for exhalation.

Human chorionic gonadotropin (hCG). A hormone produced by the trophoblast cells, which are present in early embryos and will eventually form part of the placenta. Measuring hCG levels is useful for identifying a normal pregnancy, detecting pathological pregnancies, and monitoring hCG levels following a miscarriage or abortion.

Hysterosalpingography. A procedure where an X-ray is used to look at the uterus and fallopian tubes after injecting a dye to make them visible to see if the fallopian tubes are blocked. Also known as tubal patency test.

Hysteroscopy. A visual examination of the cervix and interior of the uterus using a special camera.

In vitro fertilization (IVF). A process where eggs are taken from a woman's ovaries and fertilized by sperm in a lab. The fertilized eggs (embryos) are then put back into the woman's uterus with the hope of achieving pregnancy. It's often used by couples having trouble getting pregnant naturally.

Intrauterine insemination (IUI). Also known as artificial insemination, this fertility treatment involves placing concentrated sperm directly into the uterus to help increase the chances of pregnancy. It's often the first step in treating infertility.

Laparoscopic oophorectomy. A minimally invasive surgical procedure that removes one or both ovaries through a few small incisions in the lower abdomen.

Laparoscopy. A minor surgical procedure where a small incision is made, typically near the belly button, to insert a camera for visual inspection and possible surgical intervention within the abdominal area.

Lymphedema. A condition where excess fluid collects in tissues and causes swelling, usually in the arms or legs.

Molar pregnancy. A rare type of pregnancy complication where the tissue that normally becomes a fetus instead becomes an abnormal growth.

Papillary mesothelioma of the peritoneum. Also known as well-differentiated papillary mesothelioma (WDPM). An uncommon type of cancer that affects the protective linings of various organs. It can appear in the lining of the abdomen (known as the peritoneum), the lining around the lungs (called the pleura), or around the testicles (known as the tunica vaginalis). This cancer is characterized by the formation of small, nipple-like structures on the affected tissues.

Polycystic ovary syndrome (PCOS). A chronic hormonal condition that affects women of reproductive age and can cause cysts to develop on the ovaries.

Preeclampsia. A serious health issue that can happen in the later stages of pregnancy. It involves a sudden rise in blood pressure, excessive weight gain, swelling, protein in urine, severe headaches, and trouble with vision. If it isn't treated, it can lead to a more dangerous condition called eclampsia.

Rh-negative. Lacking the Rh factor, a protein on the surface of red blood cells.

RhoGAM (Rho(D) immune globulin). An injectable medication that prevents Rhesus (Rh) incompatibility during pregnancy.

Sonogram. An image from an ultrasound.

Triploidy. A rare condition where a cell has 69 total chromosomes instead of 46. This condition causes severe health problems for the fetus, often leading to miscarriage or early infant death.

Tubal patency test. A test to discover if the fallopian tubes are blocked. Also known as hysterosalpingography.

Ultrasound. A diagnostic medical procedure that uses two-dimensional images to enable examination of organs, tissues, and blood flow without the need for incisions. It is commonly used in obstetrics for monitoring fetal development and detecting abnormalities during pregnancy.

To learn more about Jami Crist and her other ongoing projects, click the QR Code below:

Printed in the USA
CPSIA information can be obtained
at www.ICGtesting.com
LVHW092144221024
794573LV00004B/26